The Eight-Step Approach to Teaching Clinical Nursing

SECOND EDITION

The Eight-Step Approach to Teaching Clinical Nursing

TOOLS FOR NURSE EDUCATORS

SECOND EDITION

Lydia R. Zager, MSN, RN, NEA-BC
Co-Executive Director, Leading Learning LLC
Clinical Professor, College of Nursing, University of South Carolina
Educational Consultant
Columbia, South Carolina

Loretta Manning, MSN, RN, GNP
President, I CAN Publishing®, Inc.
Co-Executive Director, Leading Learning LLC
Educational Consultant
Duluth, Georgia

JoAnne Herman, PhD, RN
Professor Emerita, College of Nursing, University of South Carolina
Columbia, South Carolina

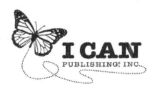

I CAN Publishing®, Inc. ◆ Duluth, GA
www.icanpublishing.com

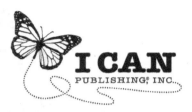

The publisher is dedicated to provide competent and reliable information regarding the subject matter covered. However, it is sold with the understanding that the authors and publisher are not engaged in rendering legal or other professional advice. Nurse Practice Acts often vary from state to state and if legal or other expert assistance is required, the services of a professional should be sought. The authors and publisher specifically disclaim any liability that is incurred from the use or application of the contents of this book.

ISBN: 978-0-9903542-4-6

Library of Congress Control Number: 2016958926

Printed in the United States of America
Second Edition

Copies of this book may be obtained from:

I CAN Publishing®, Inc.
2650 Chattahoochee Drive, Suite 100
Duluth, GA 30097
770.495.2488
www.icanpublishing.com

Cover Design: Teresa R. Davidson, Greensboro, NC
Interior Design: Mary Jo Zazueta, Traverse City, MI
Publishing Service Manager: Jennifer Robinson, Duluth, GA
Editorial Assistant: Larry Zager, MSN, Columbia, SC

Contents

Contributors

Thank you to the following nursing professionals who contributed to the content of this book.

Kate K. Chappell, MSN, APRN, CPNP-PC
Clinical Associate Professor
College of Nursing
University of South Carolina
Columbia, South Carolina

Cristy DeGregory, PhD, RN Gerontologist
Clinical Assistant Professor
College of Nursing
University of South Carolina
Columbia, South Carolina

Kimberly Glenn, MN, RN, CPN
Clinical Professor Emerita
College of Nursing
University of South Carolina
Columbia, South Carolina

Eileen Leaphart, MN, RNC, RTSC
Clinical Professor Emerita
College of Nursing
University of South Carolina
Columbia, South Carolina

Erin M. McKinney, MN, RNC, CHSE
Clinical Professor Emerita
Director, Clinical Simulation Lab
College of Nursing
University of South Carolina
Columbia, South Carolina

Heather Schneider, MSN, RN-BC
Clinical Assistant Professor
College of Nursing
University of South Carolina
Columbia, South Carolina

Ellen Synovec, MN, RN, NEA-BC
Clinical Professor Emerita
College of Nursing
University of South Carolina
Columbia, South Carolina

Preface

*"We often think of nursing as giving meds on time, checking an X-ray to see
if the doctor needs to be called, or taking an admission at 2:00 a.m. with a smile
on our faces. Too often, we forget all the other things that make our job what
it truly is: caring and having a desire to make a difference."*

~ Erin Pettengill, Missionary Nurse through Mission to the World (MTW)

Clinical nursing education is as important today as it has always been for student success and to help ensure our students can provide safe quality care to their clients. Today's expectations for the new graduates after passing the NCLEX® are to practice as if they have been working for a year! At the same time, opportunities for clinical sites are diminishing. Nursing schools are challenged to find excellent clinical experiences that help students integrate what they know while developing competent clinical skills so they are able to provide safe and effective care.

Simulation has become one of the answers to these challenges. One might think that simulation is an easy way to replace clinical, but for those of you currently using simulation, you know it takes a lot of time to develop and run scenarios that meet the educational and practice standards required for our students. During our consultations and faculty workshops across the country, there has been an identified need to provide additional information to guide faculty through this maze in linking nursing standards to simulation.

We are pleased to include in this second edition of *The Eight-Step Approach to Teaching Clinical Nursing* two new chapters on simulation. We have guest authors for the two chapters: Erin McKinney, Director Client Simulation Lab and Kate K. Chappell, Clinical Associate Professor. Both of these clinical faculty were part of the National Council of State Boards of Nursing Simulation Study at the College of Nursing at the University of South Carolina, which was a designated study site. They are both experts in designing and running scenarios and have been instrumental in adding simulation to every clinical course, both at the undergraduate and graduate level.

Engaging the Learner Activities for students is another new feature in this second edition. They are included at the end of each chapter. These student-centered learning activities will assist you with engaging the students in their own learning, connecting classroom to clinical, and reflecting and linking NCLEX® standards to practice. The activities can be tailored for clinical, lab, simulation, and the classroom. The activities refer students to the books *The Eight-Step Approach to Student Clinical Success* (Zager, Manning, Herman, 2017), *Concepts Made Insanely Easy for Clinical Nursing! A New Approach to Prioritizing Clinical Nursing* (Manning & Zager, 2014), and *Medical Surgical Nursing Concepts Made Insanely Easy!* (Manning & Zager, 2014).

The second edition of *The Eight-Step Approach to Teaching Clinical Nursing* continues to honor your requests for a practical, how-to approach to clinical teaching. We want to provide you with the tools and strategies needed to begin teaching clinical nursing on day one and proceed to the last day and final clinical evaluations.

Schools continue to report they have an increasing number of new adjunct clinical instructors as nursing faculty retire. Rarely do nursing instructors get any formal preparation in education and teaching. Orientation to the role of clinical instructor varies greatly from school to school. New clinical instructors are often expert clinicians, but need preparation for their new role as a clinical instructor. Since clinical instructors play a pivotal role in connecting theory and standards to practice, it is imperative to assist them to maximize student learning in clinical.

There are two ways you can approach this book. Our first recommendation is to read the book in its entirety for continuity of content and a complete picture of the clinical teaching process. Another approach, to expedite your learning, is to use it as a refresher and refer directly to the area where you need assistance. We hope this book will facilitate your transition into your clinical educator role and make this a positive experience if you are a new educator. If you are an experienced clinical nursing instructor, we hope the clinical tools will continue to assist you in guiding students' success, both on the NCLEX® and in clinical practice and be a resource as you mentor new clinical instructors. The tools and information have been developed from our years of clinical experience teaching nursing students nationally in a variety of academic and clinical settings.

We hope that this second edition will continue to be a useful guide and resource for you. We dedicate this work to the many nursing faculty who are busy teaching clinical nursing and are constantly striving for an increased level of excellence as a clinical instructor! We wish you much success on your journey!

Acknowledgments

We want to acknowledge and express our appreciation to the clinical faculty at the University of South Carolina in Columbia, South Carolina. We appreciate your contributions, helpful suggestions, and the adaptation and use of many of the forms in this book throughout the clinical courses.

We also want to thank nursing students across the country for their useful feedback, which has assisted us throughout the development of the tools and book.

✦ We want to thank Lydia's husband, Larry, for his insight and assistance with editing and never-ending love and support of this second edition of our book.

✦ We want to thank Loretta's husband, Randy, for his ongoing support, love, and wonderful sense of humor as we continue to juggle family, business, travel, and creating.

✦ We want to thank JoAnne's husband, Wayne, for his enthusiastic support during our writing sessions.

✦ We want to thank Jennifer Robinson, our Administrative Director, who supports us with all aspects of writing, publishing, and distributing our books; keeping us organized; and yet, at the same time, keeps us laughing to make the process enjoyable!

✦ We want to thank Mary Jo Zazueta, our friend and book designer, who always makes our work look good!

✦ We want to thank all of our contributors who add to the quality and usefulness of our book.

✦ A special thanks to our guest authors, Erin McKinney and Kate Chappell, for their excellent and timely chapters on simulation ... well done!

The Eight-Step Approach to Teaching Clinical Nursing

SECOND EDITION

Clinical Teaching: What I Need to Start

> ## IN THIS CHAPTER YOU WILL:
>
> → Assess your readiness to be a clinical instructor
>
> → Discover how your novice students think and learn
>
> → Explore the characteristics of your novice student learners
>
> → Engage multi-generational learners
>
> → Formulate teaching strategies for multi-generational learners

ASSESS YOUR READINESS TO BE A CLINICAL INSTRUCTOR

As a clinical instructor, you are one of the most important and powerful people in preparing new nurses for the future. Through a collaborative partnership with your students in clinical, you can make learning a positive experience that will set the tone for how students approach client care.

Clinical teaching can be a scary process, but not when you are adequately prepared. Through adequate preparation, clinical teaching is extremely rewarding (Koharchnik & Jakub, 2014). This chapter will help you assess your readiness to be a clinical instructor. The **Clinical Instructor Self-Assessment Questionnaire** (Refer to Appendix A) found at the end of this chapter will help you with this process as you begin your role. If the answer to any of the questions is "No," the resource column will help you find the information you need. Once you have completed your self-assessment, the next step is to understand how your novice and multi-generational students think and learn, so you can best plan and implement their clinical learning experiences.

DISCOVER HOW YOUR NOVICE STUDENTS THINK AND LEARN

The brain is structured in neural-networks. Learning is the process of developing new and more complex neuro networks. Learning is enhanced when students are actively engaged with the content through repetition and participate in the experience (Kaufer, 2016). New learning is stored in the brain with very few interconnections to other knowledge. Interconnections are formed through repetition thus connecting the new knowledge to existing knowledge. This is why novice students do not remember content from previous courses. There was no repetition or connections to existing knowledge. As an expert nurse, you are able to reach clinical decisions very quickly. You have an almost infinite number of interconnections with stored knowledge because of your extensive experience. The novice learner, your student, has minimal interconnections.

Clinical experiences are imperative in the development of the novice student nurse. For example, every time a student inserts a Foley catheter, the relationship among the steps of the procedure, sterile technique, rationale for the Foley, potential complications, and needed client teaching increase the strength of the connection of these parts to each other, resulting in an increased competence and confidence of the student (Benner, 2001).

EXPLORE THE CHARACTERISTICS OF YOUR NOVICE STUDENT LEARNERS

+ They make decisions quickly before thinking about all of the possible options, in other words, they will jump to conclusions.

+ They have difficulty applying classroom content to clinical situations.

+ They are easily overwhelmed by data (i.e., information in the medical record).

+ They have difficulty distinguishing relevant from irrelevant information.

+ They have low tolerance for ambiguity—the students just want you to tell them what to do!

+ They may be unwilling to engage in challenging problems.

+ They want to rely heavily on known solutions.

+ They often have a non-systematic approach to clinical problems.

In addition, your novice student learner approaches clinical often in a very apprehensive way. They see clinical as a set of tasks that must be accomplished. Each clinical day is a test of their personal capabilities.

So imagine their stress level! This is why establishing a positive learning environment for students is so important (Kaufer, 2016). Learning in a negative environment is very difficult. Creating a positive atmosphere during clinical maximizes learning. This does not mean that you do not correct undesired behaviors, but that feedback is done in a positive, constructive manner.

While clinical can be anxiety-producing to both the clinical instructor and students, it can also be fun. Students today thrive in an environment where they have a meaningful partnership with their clinical instructor. They want to know their instructor is a partner in their learning. Interactive Clinical Teaching Strategies (Appendix B) and the Engaging the Learner Activities at the end of each chapter provide you examples of ways to partner with students in active-learning activities that are fun and engaging.

ENGAGE THE MULTI-GENERATIONAL LEARNER

When you combine the characteristics of a novice learner with the characteristics of Generations Y and Z, it is apparent that we cannot teach current students the way we were taught. Generational differences in characteristics, values, and learning styles are a challenge for clinical instructors when we realize our old methods of teaching may need an update. Often, the majority of clinical instructors are Baby Boomers and Generation X, but the majority of your students will be Generations Y (Millennial) and Z, depending on your population.

Generations Y and Z are culturally diverse. They want balance in life and they like informality and to have fun. They are highly independent and good problem solvers, but require frequent feedback. They have been raised with high expectations that can lead to unrealistic perceptions of themselves and their clinical instructors (Nevid, 2011). The students want to know why they need to learn "this." They prefer concrete, specific information. Generations Y and Z desire personal interaction with the clinical instructor and want to be a partner in the learning process.

They are technologically literate, creative, and grew up multi-tasking—talking on the cell phone while working on the computer, and doing their homework. However, it is impossible to think about more than one thing at a time. In fact, what they do is toggle back and forth between the subjects. The danger is students then have difficulty learning anything in depth. It is a challenge for clinical instructors to help students turn off their toggle switch, so they can critically think in order to make appropriate clinical decisions.

FORMULATE TEACHING STRATEGIES FOR MULTI-GENERATIONAL LEARNERS

There are important teaching strategies that clinical instructors need in developing partnerships for learning with multi-generational learners, particularly with Generations Y and Z students. The word **COACH** can help clinical instructors successfully work with them.

C – Collaborate and Create Partnerships
O – Off with the Toggle Switch
A – Acquire Basic Knowledge
C – Communicate
H – Have to Give Frequent Feedback

C – COLLABORATE AND CREATE PARTNERSHIPS

As a clinical instructor you can create a positive clinical learning environment. Learning occurs best in an environment that feels safe and trusting to the student. This environment can be created by clinical instructors in numerous ways: treating students with respect and equitably; speaking in a calm, controlled voice; returning clinical papers in a timely manner; and giving frequent feedback in a constructive way. There are many other ways, but all of these help establish a trusting partnership between you and your students.

Generations Y and Z do not view the instructor as the only one with all of the information. They respect the clinical instructor as an expert, but they want you to partner with them in the learning process. It is still the responsibility of the clinical instructor to set expectations, adhere to standards of practice and safety; but it is not okay to be authoritarian or demeaning. You can say what you mean and mean what you say, but it is never okay to be mean. The students expect to be respected as learners and want to be included in the decisions about their learning. These decisions include: being able to make choices, ask questions, express opinions, and challenge "Why are we doing it this way?" without fear of retribution. Rather than viewing questions as a threat to you as a clinical instructor, this is an excellent opportunity to introduce or reinforce evidence-based practice. Strong interpersonal skills are essential for successful partnerships.

O – OFF WITH THE TOGGLE SWITCH

Generations Y and Z students are adept with multi-tasking, however multi-tasking is the toggling between one activity to another at a very rapid pace. Generations Y and Z's ability to text, edit a document, and post pictures on Instagram—all from their cell phones while they are doing their concept map—is impressive. With so many distracters competing for our students' attention, strategies for turning off the "toggle switch" and focusing on one topic in depth is imperative (Willis, 2006). Their ability to access large amounts of information is a great skill to have, but unfortunately this can be overwhelming. Clinical instructors need to help students prioritize what is important. The following strategies will be reviewed in detail in subsequent chapters.

- ✦ Set clear expectations for clinical performance
- ✦ Establish a structure for clinical
- ✦ Teach priority client care
- ✦ Repetition, repetition, repetition
- ✦ Use inquiry and reflection questions
- ✦ Model thinking strategies

These strategies will encourage critical thinking beyond the knowledge level to develop the clinical reasoning and judgment skills required of nurses today.

A – ACQUIRE THE KNOWLEDGE

Clinical Reasoning, which includes critical thinking, prioritization, and judgment, is the desired skill for students in clinical. However, you cannot think about nothing, so it is essential that students acquire the base knowledge they need. Knowledge acquisition begins in the classroom, but the true learning occurs when it is applied in clinical. In essence, clinical is the "flipped classroom" in nursing education. The clinical instructor is charged with connecting knowledge from the classroom to clinical. This is observed through the students' ability to construct a concept map, skill in assessing, prioritizing nursing interventions, recognizing trends and changes in the client's condition and intervening as necessary, administering medications, implementing procedures, and following and verifying the appropriateness and/or accuracy of the healthcare provider's orders.

While students have grown up with advancing technology, such as tablets and smart phones, their use of this technology has been primarily for social networking (Williams, 2015). Now they need to learn how to use this technology to acquire essential knowledge needed to give safe and effective care that is based on sound clinical reasoning that achieves desired outcomes. The use of smart phones in clinical and the availability of eBooks allow the students to have instant access to needed information. Clinical instructors need to instill in the students the desire to seek current, evidence-based information. An example is to teach students how to access discipline-specific databases, such as CINAHL® or MEDLINE®, versus just seeking information through the Internet. Creativity, such as the strategies described in the chart **Interactive Clinical Teaching Strategies** (Refer to Appendix B) and the **Engaging the Learner Activities** at the end of each chapter, can help instill the desire for students to be fully engaged in the learning process.

C – COMMUNICATE

Generations Y and Z tend to communicate cryptically because of their extensive time spent on electronic communication. Their preference is to text and use images. They have been text messaging, snap chatting, Tweeting and Twittering, etc. with family, friends, and people from different countries through smartphone and social media (Williams, 2015). However, this is very different than interpersonal communication from one person to another in the same room! This can be as simple as how to address different generations, for example, the need to address elderly clients formally with Mr. or Ms. or Sir; to being able to relate informally with Generations Y and Z clients. Knowledge of interpersonal as well as therapeutic communication skills by students will make a significant difference in their ability to establish rapport with clients and the healthcare team.

Strategies to help students improve their communication skills are very important. Here are some suggestions to use during clinical:

+ Interactive role-playing and practice

+ Interpretation of non-verbal client behaviors

✦ Role modeling appropriate therapeutic communication

✦ Feedback about student interactions with clients

✦ Simulation scenarios on effective communication

✦ Understanding cultural differences

Communication is an essential skill, best learned in clinical or in simulation. Communication impacts the therapeutic relationship the students have with their clients and is a major factor in patient safety.

H – HAVE TO GIVE FREQUENT FEEDBACK

Generations Y and Z are at home in a technological world. Generation Z grew up with smartphones where social media was always a part of their life. Both generations grew up with interactive computer games, iPods, MySpace, and expect immediate feedback about how they are doing. Without frequent feedback, students have difficulty proceeding in the learning process or will incorrectly assume they are right. As a Baby Boomer or Generation X clinical instructor, it is very easy for there to be a difference in perception between you and the student about their performance. The student may perceive the information as they just need to adjust or you were just having a conversation; but you as the clinical instructor meant this is not correct or acceptable, and the student needs to change behaviors immediately. Generations Y and Z need explicit feedback on exactly what you as the clinical instructor want to happen. It cannot be left to interpretation. Feedback and/or counseling needs to be stated and written with clear consequences if the behavior does not change.

It is very important for clinical instructors to communicate to students when they can expect to receive feedback. Equally, if not more important, is to give positive feedback to the students about what they are doing well. Mid-semester and final evaluations are not adequate to meet the needs of Generations Y and Z where instant feedback is expected. For specific strategies about providing feedback, see Chapter 7, **Assessment and Evaluation**.

Today's generation of students see learning as a social activity. Clinical provides an optimal opportunity to capitalize on team work. Working with students in pairs is a very effective way to help the novice clinical student gain confidence as they rely on each other's strengths and knowledge. Clinical instructors can encourage the students to work together when they need to problem solve. Learning how to build cohesive teams in clinical is very important as peer support is a major variable in positive job satisfaction and patient safety when they enter the workforce.

The most effective way to learn is through active engagement with the content. This is true of both knowledge and psychomotor skills. The clinical instructor's role is to create an environment where the students must independently find the information and make decisions about how that information would be applied in clinical. As novices learn, they just want you to tell them the answer. Because they are novice learners, this is going to take reinforcement and role-modeling by the clinical instructor ... you have to resist just giving them the answer, so they can begin to learn on their own. Clinical and/or simulation are the perfect place for reinforcement to occur.

Simulation, like clinical, is an excellent active-learning environment. It is an opportunity to connect the nursing concepts learned in the classroom to clinical learning and fully engage students. The interactive clinical-teaching strategies listed in Appendix B and the Engaging the Learner Activities at the end of each chapter are other ways you can engage your students in active learning.

The characteristics of the novice multi-generational learner need to be considered in all aspects of clinical and simulation (i.e., observing care given, providing feedback, questioning and evaluating student performance, etc.). The following chapters provide strategies that you can use to help your novice multi-generational nursing student be successful and give you the tools necessary to be an even better clinical instructor.

APPENDIX A

CLINICAL INSTRUCTOR SELF-ASSESSMENT QUESTIONNAIRE

Self-Assessment Questions	Yes, I Know	No, I Need Help	Resources: Where to Find Help
1. Do I understand the expected student learning outcomes of this clinical?			Refer to course syllabus and course coordinator.
2. Do I have the knowledge, skills and abilities to assist my students in the types of client care that they will give?			1. Refer to course textbooks. 2. Get clinical experience with similar types of clients. 3. Work with another experienced instructor.
3. Have I oriented to the clinical setting where I will have students? This information should include: staffing, policies and procedures, medication protocols, documentation, supply systems, equipment, safety, and quality-assurance concerns.			1. Spend time in the clinical setting prior to bringing students to clinical. 2. Review unit and clinical facility's policies and procedures. 3. Determine orientation and access requirements needed for medication, documentation and supply systems. 4. Review how to safely operate equipment used on the unit. 5. Determine what orientation is required for the students per unit protocol. 6. Discuss with the nurse manager the safety and quality monitors being evaluated.
4. Do I know what the clinical setting offers as learning opportunities for my students?			1. Meet with coordinator at the clinical site and the unit managers where the students will be. 2. Meet with other specialties areas at the clinical site as appropriate (i.e., OR, ED, etc.)
5. Do I know how to prepare the clinical staff and clients for students?			Refer to Chapter 2
6. Do I know how to prepare students by establishing the expectations and structure for the clinical day? This should include: a. orientation to the unit b. the clinical day routine c. documentation d. administer medications e. written plans for care f. pre and post conference			Refer to Chapter 2

CLINICAL INSTRUCTOR SELF-ASSESSMENT QUESTIONNAIRE *(cont'd)*

Self-Assessment Questions	Yes, I Know	No, I Need Help	Resources: Where to Find Help
7. Do I know how novice and generation Y and Z students learn and do I know how to apply teaching strategies appropriately?			Refer to Chapters 1, 2, and 3
8. Do I know how to use standards of care, (i.e., nursing practice, patient safety and NCLEX® activities) to organize my teaching?			Refer to Chapter 8
9. Do I know how to ask inquiry and reflection questions?			Refer to Chapter 3
10. Do I know how to effectively use a concept map in clinical?			Refer to Chapter 4
11. Do I know how to help students make clinical judgments through the use of thinking strategies?			Refer to Chapter 3
12. Do I know how to use interactive and innovative teaching strategies in clinical?			Refer to Chapters 1, 5, and 6; and to the Engaging the Learner Activities at the end of each chapter
13. Do I know how to give constructive feedback with a documented plan for performance improvement in clinical?			Refer to Chapter 7
14. Do I know how to do counseling for failure to meet clinical requirements?			Refer to Chapter 7
15. Do I know how to evaluate students' clinical performance?			Refer to Chapter 7
16. Do I know how to assist with simulation for my students?			Refer to Chapters 5 and 6

APPENDIX B

INTERACTIVE CLINICAL TEACHING STRATEGIES

Game	Description	Use
Scavenger Hunt	• Work in groups of 2 or 3. • Locate items on a unit and describe their exact location. • Each group will take the others to the location.	• Helpful during clinical and simulation orientation to identify location of essential equipment, supplies.
Skill Day	• A planned clinical day for clinical skill reinforcement (See Chapters 5 and 6).	• Can use early each semester to review new, previously learned and/or practice clinical skills.
Infection Control Day	• A planned day in the lab for students to identify for each client, the appropriate personal protective equipment that would need to be used in the care of the client (i.e., students are given a card to give an IM injection and must select the correct PPE, etc.).	• Assists in reinforcing infection control application that is very difficult for students to master. • Thes are important Safety and NCLEX® Standards.
Clinical Scene Investigation–CSI	• Identify a mystery, unknown clinical fact, and/or dilemma such as "why is the client suddenly itching?" • With your assistance, have the student(s) generate a list of possible explanations, such as drug-drug interactions, allergy, contact dermatitis, etc. • Next have the student(s) investigate the different explanations until they arrive at a conclusion, or realize they do not have enough data to solve the mystery.	• Helps students seek out needed information. • Helpful tool for group learning. • (Hint: This is a great strategy when the student does not know the answer!)
Deck of Doom	• Card game that reviews a clinical situation on a card. • Give a card to the student. • The student has to answer and report back to the group at post conference. • An example may include the following: The client's blood sugar at 1 PM is 47; what are the priority nursing interventions for this client?	• Post conference game, or to be used for fun during the clinical day. • Use to reinforce learning, such as hard-to-remember concepts, like the onset, peak times of different insulins. • Use in the classroom for new information or test review.

INTERACTIVE CLINICAL TEACHING STRATEGIES *(cont'd))*

Game	Description	Use
Leading Learning for the Day	• A nursing student is paired with another student to assist with clinical learning. The student leader can be assigned to a group of students.	• Helpful confidence builder. • Helps develop leadership, teambuilding and collaboration skills. • Helpful to use when the clinical situation is very busy. • Beneficial exercise during senior semesters.
War Stories	• Clinical instructors or students share clinical experiences that can be positive or negative or even funny. • Who can tell the best story?	• Connections between reality-based practice with theoretical learning. • Stories are a vivid personal teaching method that students can connect to clinical. • Stories may involve both positive and negative clinical experiences. • Ice breaker for a new clinical groups. • Serves as a bonding experience among the clinical group and the clinical instructor. • A reflection exercise for the end of the semester.
Who Wants to be a Super Nurse?	• When asking students questions in a group about information that they are expected to know (i.e., during medication administration, give them the choice of life lines to answer the question). • They can answer the question themselves. • They can ask another student (call a friend). • They can ask the group (poll the audience) and choose to agree or disagree with the answer.	• This is a great strategy to reduce the tension. • Preserves dignity of the student. • Reinforces content while still holding the students accountable for their learning. • For example, can be used prior to medication administration, procedures, post-conference and/or in the classroom.

ENGAGING THE LEARNER ACTIVITIES

STUDENT-CENTERED LEARNING ACTIVITIES
LINKED TO PROFESSIONAL AND NCLEX® STANDARDS

Resources Needed for Activity	The Eight-Step Approach for Teaching Clinical Nursing (Zager, Manning & Herman, 2017)	The Eight-Step Approach for Student Clinical Success (Zager, Manning & Herman, 2017)
Standards	**Faculty Instructions**	**Student Instructions**
Management of Care Recognize limitations of self and others and seek assistance.	**Self-Assessment Questionnaire** (Refer to Chapter 1 of *The Eight-Step Approach for Student Clinical Success*) 1. Have students complete the Self-Assessment Questionnaire. a. Identify what they perceive will be their greatest challenges. b. Identify what they perceive are their strengths. c. Share ideas about what they can do to prepare for clinical (i.e., resources, references, etc.). d. Identify specific learning goals they have for themselves.	**Self-Assessment Questionnaire** (Refer to Chapter 1) 1. Complete the Self-Assessment questionnaire. a. Identify your greatest challenges. b. Identify your strengths. c. Share ideas about what you can do to prepare for clinical (i.e., resources, references, etc.). d. Identify specific learning goals for yourself.
Management of Care Organize workload to manage time effectively.	**Scavenger Hunt** (Refer to Appendix B) 2. Conduct the Scavenger Hunt the first day of clinical to help students learn where items are located on the unit where they are assigned.	**Scavenger Hunt** (Refer to the Scavenger Hunt at the end of Chapter 1) 2. Look for the items on the Scavenger Hunt and write where they are located on your assigned unit.
Assessing Your Learning Style	**Characteristics of Novice and Multi-Generational Learner** (Refer the students to Chapter 1 of *The Eight-Step Approach for Student Clinical Success*) 3. Have the students: a. Identify characteristics of a novice learner that apply to them. b. Identify which generational characteristics apply to them. c. Identify strategies that can help them be successful in their learning.	**Characteristics of Novice and Multi-Generational Learner** (Refer to Chapter 1) 3. Review in Chapter 1 the characteristics of a novice and multi-generational learner. a. Identify characteristics of a novice learner that apply to you. b. Identify which generational characteristics apply to you. c. Identify strategies that can help you be successful in your learning.

CHAPTER 2

Structuring the Clinical Day

IN THIS CHAPTER YOU WILL LEARN ABOUT:

- → Structuring the clinical day
- → Structuring how students organize their clinical findings
- → Structuring medication administration

STRUCTURING THE CLINICAL DAY

Many new clinical instructors feel overwhelmed with how to organize a clinical day. The thought of coordinating eight to ten nursing students with medication administration alone can result in a sleepless night. Our goal is to provide you with tools to assist you in planning, structuring, and organizing the clinical day. Structure is essential for learning, particularly with novice generation Y and Z learners (Benner, 2001; Nevid, 2011).

A step often left out is preparing the unit staff for the students. Good communication with the staff can make all the difference in the quality of the clinical experience and the relationships among the staff, you, and the students. Share with the staff the course syllabus, student learning objectives, skills the students cannot perform without you, and skills students can do with the nursing staff. Determine how you will communicate student clinical assignments and what aspects of client care students will be performing. Share this information with the staff while you are orienting to the unit.

The next step is to plan your clinical day. **Appendix A (How to Structure a Typical Clinical Day)** provides an example of how to structure a typical clinical day. When you are working with novice nursing students, they need structure to decrease their anxiety and optimize their learning experience. **How to Structure a Typical Clinical Day** (Appendix A) can be adapted to your clinical setting. It may seem like a lot of work, but the time spent in planning will help ensure the clinical day is organized, which contributes to both yours and your students' success.

STRUCTURING HOW STUDENTS ORGANIZE THEIR CLINICAL FINDINGS

Students are overwhelmed with how to organize the information they get from report and from orders for procedures and medications. Without a structured format, students can be disorganized in their thinking, delivery of care, and their ability to document accurately. **Typical Day Schedule: A Student Guide** (Appendix B) and description of a **Shift Report Using SBAR Format** (Appendix C) can be extremely useful to the students. It helps them organize their clinical day and give an effective and accurate report.

These tools can be very effective when shared with the students during the clinical orientation. The tools will help students understand the expectations for clinical performance, document with accuracy, and most importantly, provide safe and effective care in a timely manner.

STRUCTURING MEDICATION ADMINISTRATION

Developing a medication-administration practice that incorporates current guidelines for safe medication administration is essential. Adverse drug events, when harm is caused by a medication error, affect approximately 5% of hospitalized clients and are the most common type of inpatient error (Agency for Healthcare Research and Quality, 2015). Multiple federal agencies—Agency for Healthcare Research and Quality (AHRQ), Institute for Safe Medication (ISMP), Quality and Safety Education for Nurses (QSEN) etc.—have developed guidelines designed to decrease medication errors.

As a clinical instructor you are obligated to help students develop a medication practice that incorporates medication safety guidelines. These guidelines include elements that are particularly important when teaching students how to administer medications; such as to establish a no-interruption zone and use a structured checklist for medication administration that includes supplies and clinical information needed prior to giving medications (Beyea, 2014). The **Medication Administration Protocol: A Safe Approach** (Appendix D) incorporates the recommended guidelines for safe medication administration. It is important that you know the unit and institutional guidelines for medication administration and documentation so you can be in compliance before you bring your students to clinical.

When clinical instructors consistently use a structured process, students develop safe medication administration habits essential to prevent medication errors. The medication protocol helps students administer medications safely and efficiently, and it provides you confidence that the students are prepared to give their medications.

In order for the medication protocol to have the maximum effect, it should be implemented across all clinical courses in the curriculum. This prevents students from having to learn a new structure for giving medications with each clinical instructor. This consistency throughout the courses provides repetition and strengthens the safe medication administration habit for the students. The process for giving medications should not be interrupted as it is one of the leading causes of medication errors (Beyea, 2014). Questions should be asked before beginning the process of medication administration. Do not interrupt the student with questions during the process (i.e., pulling the medications, checking the medications against the medication record and the healthcare provider's orders, etc.) except to intervene if an error is about to be made. Students need to check before giving medications if they will be giving medications with black box warnings (BBW) or any high-alert medications. Both categories of drugs can cause serious reactions or potential safety considerations (Hughes, 2008; Manning, 2017).

Structuring the clinical day, medication administration, care of the client, and pre- and post-conference are more than just being organized. It is essential to help your students provide safe quality care. Organization helps prevent omissions of care, and is necessary for the students' learning process. The students may not tell you, but they appreciate a well-organized and structured clinical day!

APPENDIX A

Chapter 2

HOW TO STRUCTURE A TYPICAL CLINICAL DAY

Time	Student Activity	Instructor Reminders and Notes (The following are examples.)
6:45 AM Prior to pre-conference	Get report (SBAR) from your nurse. Check for: • New orders • New medications • Time of 1st medication • Check if NPO for tests, surgery or procedures. If so, will they get any of their medications (i.e., insulin, anti-hypertensives, etc.)?	The goal for clinical instructor prior to the beginning of clinical is to determine: • Which student, which client, what skills, and what medications are going to require your attention? • How will you prioritize and guide the students in prioritizing their activities? Example: • Prioritize the student's learning needs (i.e., tracheotomy suctioning and does the student need instruction and guidance with the skill?). • Prioritize assigned client's needs (i.e., acuity, medications times; i.e., 7 AM medication). • Know the diagnostic exams (i.e., is there any prep, medications to be given, NPO status?).
Pre-conference	Review student clinical concept maps and plans for the day.	Assess if the students are prepared: • Do they have their clinical concept map with predicted client's needs and interventions that are accurate? • Get a brief SBAR report from your students. • Use inquiry questions in your assessment. • Schedule student activities that require clinical instructor supervision beginning with early AM medications and scheduled procedures.

HOW TO STRUCTURE A TYPICAL CLINICAL DAY *(cont'd))*

Time	Student Activity	Instructor Reminders and Notes (The following are examples.)
7:00 – 7:20 AM	See your client for a quick assessment: • Respiratory status, in pain, safety issues, etc. • Check IVs. Make sure they are patent and running at the right rate with the right fluid. • Check for any other lines, tubes, that they are patent, and note the drainage. • Take BP and pulse. • Check on blood sugars or obtain glucometer reading. • Administer insulin or other before meals medications. • Always check to see if the medication has been given, is being held, etc. • Prepare for any scheduled tests.	• Meet students as scheduled.
8:00 – 9:30 AM	• Give AM medications. • Perform other client procedures as ordered. • Prepare client for scheduled procedures/ surgery if scheduled. • Complete focused system-specific assessment. • Note any trending of clinical findings that could indicate potential complications. • Document findings, inform instructor and nursing staff of any concerns. • Complete or ensure AM care is done (often a good time to do the assessment).	• Use the Medication Protocol: Safe Approach. • Divide students into groups. • Have part of the students begin with medication administration. • Have part of the students complete AM care and do assessments. • Recommend doing procedures that require supervision after AM medications are given. • Note any trending signs of potential complications with your students' clients. • Elicit staff support where needed.

cont'd on next page

HOW TO STRUCTURE A TYPICAL CLINICAL DAY *(cont'd)*

Time	Student Activity	Instructor Reminders and Notes (The following are examples.)
9:30 – 10 AM	• First documentation entered to include assessments and other findings. • Implement and evaluate your priority nursing interventions (i.e., coughing and deep breathing, etc.). • "MOVE Your Client"–Ambulate, get up in chair or turn (as condition allows); assess client's activity tolerance and document (Manning, L. & Zager, L. 2014, p. 146 "The MOVE").	Begin making rounds of student's clients: • See priority or unstable clients first (i.e., clients with indwelling lines, IVs, tubes, etc.). • Facilitate students with their care. Are they meeting the priority needs of the client? • Ask students inquiry questions and/or reflection questions (see chart in Chapter 3 for suggestions).
10:30 AM	• Continue to assess client and document. • Evaluate response to PRN medications. • Complete any treatments or procedures as ordered (this may be earlier depending on the time of the test). • Complete client teaching and document. • Continue to check for new healthcare provider's orders. • Check for lab result (i.e., PTT and INR if on heparin, etc.).	• Ensure students have completed assessments, evaluations, and documentation of their client's progress toward outcomes. • Assist students with other procedures, changes in healthcare provider's orders as needed, etc.
11:00 – 12:00	• Give medications as ordered. • Assist with meals as needed. • Assess vital signs as ordered. • Continue to assess client and document findings. • Assess and provide care for indwelling lines, peg tubes, etc. • Continue interventions and assess effectiveness.	• Assist students as needed and evaluate if there are students who need additional guidance.
Lunch	• Plan your lunch around your client's needs (you will need to cover for your fellow students).	• Schedule the students' and your breaks and meals around client's needs. • Depending on the level of the students, i.e. if this is their first semester versus a senior nursing student, decide if they will cover for each other or go as a group.

HOW TO STRUCTURE A TYPICAL CLINICAL DAY *(cont'd)*

Time	Student Activity	Instructor Reminders and Notes (The following are examples.)
1:00 – 1:45 PM	• Continue to assess if desired client outcomes are being met and documented. • Are there any trending concerns in the client's assessment findings? If so, report to your instructor and the client's nurse. • Continue client teaching and document. • Complete any scheduled interventions or procedures.	• Continue rounds of students' clients. • Ensure students have completed their assigned care and it is documented.
1:45 – 2:30 PM	• Complete final assessment and document client's progress toward desired outcomes. • Document I & O (i.e., IV or PO intake, NG tube or Foley output, etc.). • Make sure client is safe (i.e. ,bed rails up, bed alarms in place, etc.). • Ensure the client's room is neat. • Check to see if all medications have been given and documented with client responses	• Evaluate student documentation. • Has the student documented the client's response to interventions and progress toward outcomes? • Does their documentation include changes in the client's assessment, if applicable, and what steps were taken? • Are I & O's recorded? • Are there any medications, treatments or procedures that have not been done? • Make quick rounds to ensure all clients are safe.
2:30 PM	Give SBAR to the assigned nurse.	Ensure all students have reported off using SBAR to the assigned nurse
2:30 – 3:00 PM	Attend post-conference.	Conduct post conference: use inquiry and reflection questions (i.e., what could they have delegated today, was there any particular concern about room placement, what infection control PPE was required for the care of the client, etc.)
HOME	Go home, kick your feet up and be happy another clinical day is over! Seriously: Take time to reflect on how the day went and what you can do to improve your next clinical day.	Go home and be thankful another clinical day is completed successfully. Take time to reflect on how the day went and what you can do to improve your next clinical day with your students.

APPENDIX B

TYPICAL DAY SCHEDULE: A STUDENT GUIDE
(May vary per clinical and client needs)

When you arrive, before 6:45 AM
+ Get report from your nurse.
+ Check for new orders, new meds, time of first med, check if NPO for test, which meds are they getting, AM blood sugars.

7:00 – 7:20 AM Preconference
+ Assess BP and pulse.
+ Give 7:30 meds, insulin (check to see if it has been given).
+ See your client assess quickly, check IVs, make sure they are patent and running at the right rate with the right fluid, check for any other lines, tubes that they are patent and what is draining.

By 9:30 AM
+ Give meds and complete assessment or vice versa as appropriate.
+ Enter your assessment findings in the documentation system per protocol.
+ Give AM care (a great time to do or complete your client's assessment).

10 AM
+ Document opening nursing note with AM assessment by_____(Time).

10:30 AM
+ Treatments or procedures ordered (this may come earlier if scheduled for tests).
+ Implement client teaching as needed. Continue to check for new orders from healthcare provider.
+ Check for lab results, (i.e., PTT & INR if on heparin, blood sugar if on insulin, etc.). 11:00–12:00 check for noon blood sugar if ordered, eat lunch, feed client if needed.

11 AM
+ Document vital signs, note any trending that could indicate potential complication. Continue to assess client's response and progress toward desired outcomes.

Lunch for 30 min between the hours of 11:00 and 12:00 based on your client's needs. Coordinate with other students.

Give 11 and 12 o'clock meds if ordered, flush Intermittent Access Venous Device per protocol
+ Continue to reinforce client teaching and interventions to help your client achieve the outcomes and continuously reassess your client.

1:00 PM
+ Wrap-up, do final assessment, make sure the client is safe, needs are met, and the room is neat and free of clutter.
+ Complete I & O, document per protocol. Check to see that all meds have been given and documented.

1:30 PM
+ Document your final notes: include evaluation of your client's progress or lack of progress toward the desired outcomes.
+ Is your client getting better? Include I & O. Document information as appropriate on IV flow rates, insertion sites, drains, dressings, etc. Document client teaching and evaluation of client's level of understanding.

By 2:00 PM
+ Report off to your nurse and your clinical instructor using SBAR.

2:00 PM Post-conference

SHIFT REPORT USING SBAR FORMAT

The Situation and Background will only need to be entered the first time you report on this client.

Situation: Client Name, Age, Sex

Room Number

Healthcare Providers

Background: Admission Diagnosis (date of surgery)

Past medical history that is significant (hypertension, heart failure, etc.)

Allergies

This information should be included in each report if applicable.

Assessment: Code Status, any advance directives, DNR orders, Power of Attorney Health Care (POAHC)

Procedures done in previous 24 hours including results/outcomes (include client's post-procedure vitals/assessment)

Abnormal assessment findings

Abnormal vital signs

IV fluids/drips/site; when is site to be changed

Current pain score—what has been done to manage pain

Safety Needs—fall risk, skin risk, etc.

Recommendations: Needed changes in the plan of care (diet, activity, medication, consultations)?

What are you concerned about?

Discharge planning

Pending labs/x-rays, etc.

Calls to healthcare provider _____about_____

What the next shift needs to do or be aware of (i.e., labs to be drawn in AM, etc.)

APPENDIX D

MEDICATION ADMINISTRATION PROTOCOL: A SAFE APPROACH

Prior to Beginning Medication Administration

1. Prior to beginning medication administration:
   a. Verify orders.
   b. Gather needed client assessments (i.e., BP, pulse, or other required assessment data).
   c. Check needed lab results (i.e., potassium level if client has furosemide ordered, blood sugar or glucometer readings for insulin, drug levels like digoxin).
   d. Check to see if any clients are NPO, or are going for procedures, dialysis, etc.
   e. Check to see if any medications have Black Box Warnings or are high-alert medications.

2. Pull the Medication Record for your client (the MAR). Do only one client at a time.

3. Know the purpose of each medication. Do you have all the information you need prior to giving the medication? If not, obtain and review this information and have it ready.
   a. Action of the drug
   b. Key adverse reactions
   c. Nursing implications
   d. Why the client is getting the medication. Is the drug appropriate for this client?
   e. Food/drug or drug/drug interactions
   f. Known allergies
   g. What do you need to teach your client about the medication? (Manning & Rayfield, 2017)

4. Let your instructor know you are ready to check off your medications.
Preparing Medications for Administration
5. Obtain the medications you need. (Your clinical instructor may have to do this for you based on the medication system in your facility, i.e., Bar Code Scanners, Pyxis, etc.).
6. Have MAR visible and check your medications (i.e., vials, IV piggy backs, IV fluids, etc.) beside the ordered drug on the MAR.

7. Check the medications against the MAR in order as they are listed. Leave medications in packaging and do not draw medications from the vials without your instructor.
   a. Do you have the right medication?
   b. Is the medication scheduled for this time?
   c. Is it the right dose?
   d. Is there any information you need to document prior to giving the medication (i.e., BP readings, digoxin levels, etc.) that you do not have?
   e. Is there any medication that needs to be held or any order that needs to be questioned?
   f. Has the medication already been given?
   g. Based on what you know about the medication, does it make sense (rationale) that this client is getting this medication? (Manning & Rayfield, 2017)

8. With your instructor, prepare the correct dosage (i.e., cut the pill, draw up the correct dose from a vial for IV, IM, subcutaneous injections, etc.).
Administering the Medications
9. Once you have completed the check-off with your instructor, take your MAR and the medications still in their packaging (it may be the Bar Code Scanner or beside medication delivery system) to the client's bedside.
10. Perform seven rights for medications and check your medications with the MAR as you give the medication to the client.
11. Sign off the medications on the MAR or documentation system as the client takes them and answer any client or family questions.
12. Return the MAR to the appropriate place and note when your next medications are due. Document as appropriate.
13. Evaluate client's response to medications per protocol. (Manning & Rayfield, 2017)
14. Document client's response and progress toward outcome.

ENGAGING THE LEARNER ACTIVITIES

STUDENT-CENTERED LEARNING ACTIVITIES
LINKED TO PROFESSIONAL AND NCLEX® STANDARDS

Resources Needed for Activity	*The Eight-Step Approach for Teaching Clinical Nursing* (Zager, Manning & Herman, 2017)	*The Eight-Step Approach for Student Clinical Success* (Zager, Manning & Herman, 2017)
Standards	**Faculty Instructions**	**Student Instructions**

Management of Care
 	
Organize workload to manage time effectively.
	Typical Day Schedule Student Guide
	(Refer to end of Chapter 2 in *The Eight-Step Approach for Student Clinical Success*)
	Review how to do the schedule during orientation and review each clinical day.
	1. Have the students complete the blank template of the schedule to reflect requirements of the assigned unit.
	   a. Have students make the changes on the schedule to reflect their client's needs.
		Typical Day Schedule Student Guide
		(Refer to Chapter 2)
		
		1. Complete the blank template of the schedule to reflect the requirements of the unit you are assigned.
		   a. Change the schedule as needed each clinical day to reflect your client's needs.

Pharmacological and Parenteral Therapies
 	
Prepare and administer medication, using rights of medication administration.
	Medication Administration Protocol: A Safe Approach
	(Refer to Appendix D)
	Pair students for this exercise.
	2. Review and role model the Medication Administration Protocol: A Safe Approach.
	   a. Have students return the demonstration.
	   b. Provide feedback.
		Medication Administration Protocol: A Safe Approach
		(Refer to end of Chapter 2)
		
		2. Review the Medication Administration Protocol: A Safe Approach prior to clinical.
		   a. Demonstrate how to follow the Medication Administration Protocol: A Safe Approach.
		   b. Give feedback to your partner.

Management of Care
 	
Provide and receive report on assigned clients.
	SBAR Report
	(Refer to blank SBAR form, end of Chapter 2, in *The Eight-Step Approach for Student Clinical Success*)
	3. Review the components of the SBAR report.
	   a. Provide students with a client scenario and have them write a SBAR report
	   b. Have students give the SBAR report.
	   c. Discuss what information is and is not a priority to report.
		SBAR Report
		(Refer to blank SBAR form, end of Chapter 2)
		
		3. Review the components of the SBAR report.
		   a. Prepare a written SBAR report
		   b. Give the SBAR report.
		   c. Use the written client scenario and determine what is and is not a priority to report.

Management of Care
 	
Provide and receive report on assigned clients.
	SBAR Report—Missing Information
	4. Use the SBAR examples (Refer to *The Eight-Step Approach for Student Clinical Success*) and omit key pieces of information (i.e., VS, IV rate, lab value, etc.) from the report. Have the students identify:
	   a. Additional information needed when giving the report to the next shift.
	   b. Additional information needed when calling the healthcare provider to report a change in client's condition?
		SBAR Report—Missing Information
		4. Determine what is missing from the SBAR report.
		   a. What additional information is needed if you were giving a report to the next shift?
		   b. What additional information is needed when you are calling the healthcare provider to report a change in client's condition?

NOTES

CHAPTER 3

Improving Clinical Reasoning

IN THIS CHAPTER YOU WILL LEARN HOW TO:

- → Develop prioritization strategies
- → Apply inquiry and reflection questions
- → Use thinking strategies to develop clinical reasoning

Now that you have a structure for organizing your clinical day, a protocol for medication administration, and an example of a typical day to help students organize their care, it is time to help students improve their clinical reasoning, ability to prioritize, and ultimately their clinical judgment. When we have worked with clinical facilities, they want the new graduate nurses to have clinical reasoning skills. Observation of student performance is a part of the clinical instructor's role. However, observation does not give you information on what the student is thinking. Likewise, questions asked randomly without purpose lead to inconsistent outcomes (Koharchnik, Caputi, Robb, & Culleiton, 2015). When clinical instructors use observation with questions asked in a deliberate and systematic way, it strengthens the student's clinical reasoning skills and their ability to prioritize care.

PRIORITIZATION

Prioritization is now an expectation of the new graduate, and it is reflected in the type of questions students must answer to be successful on NCLEX®. "This competency requires a new approach to thinking and processing clinical data" (Manning & Zager, 2014, p. 11). Students must expand basic assessments to include specific elements that impact their clinical findings. Thinking strategies such as compare, contrast, and trend (Refer to Appendix E), help students develop their prioritization skills. Prioritizing care, to include who to see first, which healthcare provider order to implement first, or what medication should be administered first, are great activities to help your students gain confidence in their ability to prioritize.

In addition to prioritization, "Today's nurses are expected to know more about interpretation of clinical assessments or laboratory findings than simply the normal and abnormal ranges. To use current intravenous drugs, which must be carefully monitored and titrated, nurses need sophisticated knowledge of pharmacokinetics, hemodynamics, and cardiac function" (Benner, Sutphen, Leonard, & Day, 2010, p. 27). The next chart compares basic clinical assessments previously required to the current clinical expectations of trending for potential complications for nursing students and/or graduates based on the concept of oxygenation. This is a great exercise to do in post-conference with students as you can apply it to any concept and/or disease process.

COMPARISON OF BASIC CLINICAL ASSESSMENTS WITH TRENDING FOR POTENTIAL COMPLICATIONS

BASIC CLINICAL ASSESSMENTS	TREND FOR POTENTIAL COMPLICATIONS
Medical Diagnosis: Chronic Obstructive Pulmonary Disease	System-Specific Pathophysiology: Obstructive airflow that impedes respirations. Concept: Oxygenation (altered)
1. Respiratory Rate?	1. Respiratory Rate? • Compare, contrast, and trend from previous assessment. (i.e., shallow, nasal flaring present, etc.) • Has client just received a narcotic that may affect the breathing?
2. Breath sounds? Equality?	2. Breath sounds? Equality? • Compare, contrast, and trend from previous assessment (i.e., adventitious sounds, use of accessory muscles, etc.).
3. O_2 saturation?	3. O_2 saturation? • Is the finger cold? • Is the probe in appropriate place? • Is it connected to monitor? • Does the client have the appropriate amount of oxygen with the correct delivery system (i.e., nasal cannula, mask, etc.)? • Does the client have peripheral vascular insufficiency such as Raynaud's Disease?
4. Hypoxia?	4. Is the client presenting with **early** versus **late** signs of hypoxia? • Early: restless, increase in the HR and RR. • Late: confusion, decrease in the HR and RR.
5. Arterial blood gas values?	5. Arterial blood gas values: • Trending from previous values. • Is the client currently experiencing changes (i.e., RR, breath sounds, shallow respirations, etc.)?

COMPARISON OF BASIC CLINICAL ASSESSMENTS
WITH TRENDING FOR POTENTIAL COMPLICATIONS *(cont'd)*

BASIC CLINICAL ASSESSMENTS	TREND FOR POTENTIAL COMPLICATIONS
Medical Diagnosis: Chronic Obstructive Pulmonary Disease	System-Specific Pathophysiology: Obstructive airflow that impedes respirations. Concept: Oxygenation (altered)
6. Which client should be assessed first? (Students will often answer with any client presenting with an airway issue instead of looking at the client who needs immediate action. Use the right column to help them critically reason based on the clinical findings.)	6. Arterial blood gas values of three clients: a. A client with COPD who has RR 18/min and in one hour increased to 24/min. b. A client with COPD with RR 22/min. c. A client with asthma who had an acute exacerbation with audible wheezing 30 minutes ago. Clinical instructors: Explain to the students prioritization is more than just relying on the "ABC's" for the correct answer; now it is more complex. You must make a clinical decision based on the client that needs immediate action, which would make the correct answer client c. Option c is the answer due to client requiring immediate intervention. Options a and b are chronic with no immediate distress and Option c is an acute problem that mandates immediate assessment and/or intervention. They all have airway complications!
7. Which of these clinical assessment findings indicates a desired outcome from the nursing care for a client with COPD? (Students will often answer with the desired outcome of i.e., respiratory rate within defined limits for client. As a clinical instructor help the students critically reason through what would be a realistic expectation for a COPD client.)	7. Which of these clinical assessment findings indicate a desired outcome from the nursing care for a client with COPD? a. Client presents with clear breath sounds. b. Client presents with an O_2 sat of 94%, which increased from 86% three hours ago. c. Client with COPD participates in physical activity with no shortness of breath. Clinical instructors: Guide the students to see Options a and c are unrealistic for this client. Option b is the answer. Option b is realistic and is a desired outcome for this client with COPD. In order to answer the question, it is imperative to recognize normal findings for a client with COPD. It is not as easy as using the ABCs! It is imperative to compare and review trends in order to make a clinical decision.

Manning, L & Zager, L. (2014). Medical surgical nursing concepts made insanely easy: A new approach to prioritizing nursing! Duluth, GA: I CAN Publishing, Inc. p. 12.

SAFETY: A New Systematic Approach to Prioritize Nursing Care Based on Standards (Appendix A) is a tool for your students to use as they learn the prioritization process. This will help develop your students clinical reasoning skills as they begin to understand there can be many reasons why a client and/or a situation is a priority besides having airway and circulation issues. The priority could be a safety issue with a client who is at risk for committing suicide or it could be that the nurse needs to intervene because of standard of practice is not being followed or to question a new order from the healthcare provider. The SAFETY model is discussed in detail in

Chapter 8 with strategies on how to use it throughout clinical and the classroom. (For additional information on prioritizing concepts, refer to the book *Medical Surgical Nursing Concepts Made Insanely Easy: A New Approach to Prioritizing Nursing!* (Manning & Zager, 2014).

INQUIRY QUESTIONS

Inquiry questions require the students to reveal what they know. There is a hierarchy of inquiry questions from knowledge to synthesis. It is essential for clinical instructors to ask questions that take the student beyond memorization of facts to application, analysis, and synthesis. Asking inquiry questions helps clinical instructors determine if the student knows how to give safe and effective care (Pesut & Herman, 1999). This also helps students learn the kind of questions they need to ask themselves when the clinical instructor is not present. Begin the inquiry process with knowledge level questions:

+ Does the student know the basic facts /information about the topic?

+ If the student knows the facts, have the student apply the facts to the client's situation.

+ If the student can apply the facts to the client's situation, assist the student to make choices among options for care.

+ If the student is successful, ask questions that require the student to consider past similar clinical situations to the current one and project how the situations could apply to future clients.

Analysis and synthesis level thinking will develop as the student progresses. The following table, **Types of Inquiry Questions**, gives examples of each of these types of questions.

Types of Inquiry Questions

DEFINITIONS	EXAMPLES OF INQUIRY QUESTIONS
Knowledge: Memorized information /facts	What is the normal range for blood pressure?
Application: Connecting knowledge to a clinical situation	Which is the most important vital sign to monitor in your client who has hypertension?
Analysis: Understanding pros and cons, strengths and weaknesses or other options in decision-making	Should you administer the anti-hypertensive medication as ordered for a client who has a blood pressure of 95/60?
Synthesis: Pulling together multiple sources of experiences, data and information to make decisions about needed client care. This process may require several inquiry questions to guide the student.	What has the blood pressure been for the past two days? Is this the same or has there been a change? What could be contributing to the change in the BP? Are there any guidelines in the healthcare provider's orders regarding their BP? What are the priority nursing actions?

The Quick Approach: Inquiry Questions for Classroom and Clinical Knowledge Organized Around the "**SAFETY**" Model (Appendix A) and the SAFETY model (Refer to Chapter 8) will provide you with multiple examples of questions that you can apply in different client care situations. The questions have been written within the framework of the NCLEX-RN® activities that are based on practice and safety standards. When these questions are incorporated as you prepare the classroom exams and during clinical teaching, you will have a success formula for both clinical practice and the NCLEX-RN® for your students.

REFLECTION QUESTIONS

Reflection questions require students to think about their own thinking. Reflection challenges students to self-monitor, plan, and revise their own thinking so they can quickly self-correct (Pesut & Herman, 1999). Reflection results in safe and effective decisions about the needed client care and the prevention of complications. Reflective thinking is an essential component of clinical reasoning (Koharchnik, Caputi, Robb, & Culleiton, 2015). Clinical instructors need to role-model reflective practice and the habit of self-questioning. The way you do that is to use reflection questions. You can use **Appendix C, Example of Reflection Questions**, with your students to help them reflect on their clinical day. These questions can be used in post-conference or as an assignment due the following day. This example includes points that are a part of the **Rubric for the Concept MAP** (Refer to Chapter 4, Appendix B). Reflection questions can be changed weekly and adapted to meet the needs of the clinical day. The mark of a true professional is to reflect constantly about their clinical practice.

HOW TO USE INQUIRY AND REFLECTION QUESTIONS

Urinary Catheterization Algorithm (Appendix D) displays how clinical instructors use inquiry and reflection questions before and after a urinary catheterization. The questions included in the algorithm help the students see beyond the task to the clinical reasoning needed to provide safe and effective care even when performing procedures. Novice students without these questions will approach procedures as a task to be accomplished. Please note though, it will be important not to ask these questions during the procedure but before and after. These same types of questions apply to any procedure.

USE THINKING STRATEGIES TO DEVELOP CLINICAL REASONING

Clinical reasoning is not inherent in a novice thinker. In order to achieve this level of development in students' thinking, you need to teach them how. Role modeling is the best way (Koharchnik, Caputi, Robb, & Culleiton, 2015) to illustrate how you use clinical reasoning to make your clinical decisions. You can use inquiry and reflection questions to help students adopt a structured way of thinking about a client situation. This process will help students build clinical reasoning skills. **Thinking Strategies to Improve Students Clinical Reasoning** (Appendix E) lists thinking strategies, their definitions, and the use of them in clinical. It combines thinking strategies with inquiry and reflection questions.

APPENDIX A

Chapter 3

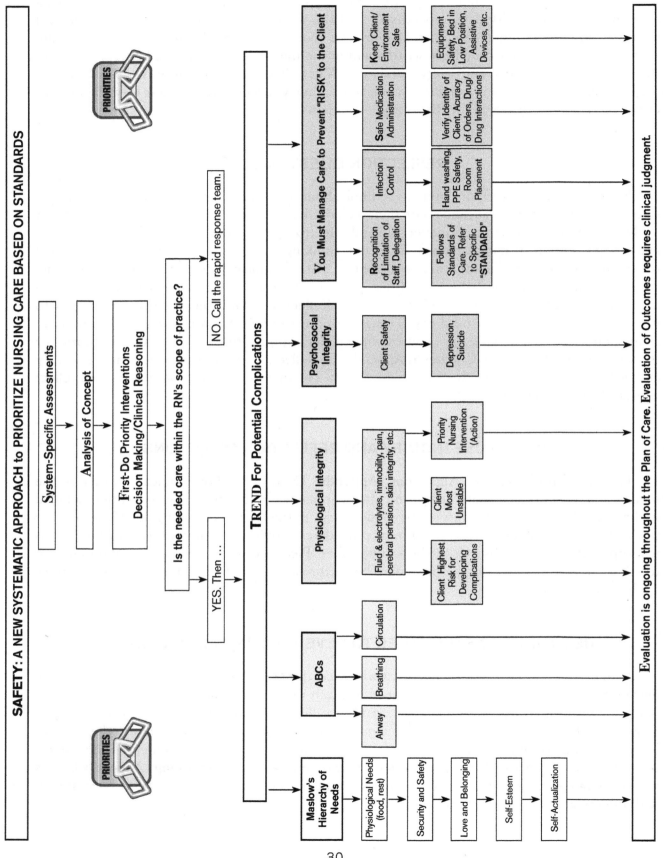

SAFETY: A NEW SYSTEMATIC APPROACH to PRIORITIZE NURSING CARE BASED ON STANDARDS

System-Specific Assessments

Analysis of Concept

First-Do Priority Interventions
Decision Making/Clinical Reasoning

Is the needed care within the RN's scope of practice?

NO. Call the rapid response team.

YES. Then ...

TREND For Potential Complications

Maslow's Hierarchy of Needs
- Physiological Needs (food, rest)
- Security and Safety
- Love and Belonging
- Self-Esteem
- Self-Actualization

ABCs
- Airway
- Breathing
- Circulation

Physiological Integrity
- Fluid & electrolytes, immobility, pain, cerebral perfusion, skin integrity, etc.
  - Client Highest Risk for Developing Complications
  - Client Most Unstable
  - Priority Nursing Intervention (Action)

Psychosocial Integrity
- Client Safety
  - Depression, Suicide

You Must Manage Care to Prevent "RISK" to the Client
- Recognition of Limitation of Staff, Delegation
  - Follows Standards of Care. Refer to Specific **"STANDARD"**
- Infection Control
  - Hand washing, PPE Safety, Room Placement
- **S**afe Medication Administration
  - Verify Identity of Client, Acuracy of Orders, Drug/ Drug Interactions
- Keep Client/ Environment Safe
  - Equipment Safety, Bed in Low Position, Assistive Devices, etc.

PRIORITIES

Evaluation is ongoing throughout the Plan of Care. Evaluation of Outcomes requires clinical judgment.

Manning, L. and Zager, L. © 2014 Medical surgical nursing concepts made insanely easy: A new approach to prioritizing nursing! Duluth, GA: I CAN Publishing, Inc. p.13.

30

THE QUICK APPROACH: INQUIRY QUESTIONS FOR CLASSROOM AND CLINICAL KNOWLEDGE ORGANIZED AROUND THE "SAFETY" MODEL
(Adapted from the 2015 RN Practice Analysis)

SYSTEM-SPECIFIC PATHOPHYSIOLOGY

1. Which of these clinical assessment findings indicate a complication with the pathophysiology related to a **Specific Disease** (acute or chronic)?

2. Which of these statements made by **the nurse, client, or family** indicates an understanding of the pathophysiology for a client diagnosed with a **Specific Disease** (acute or chronic)?

SYSTEM-SPECIFIC ASSESSMENTS

1. Which vital sign assessments would be the highest priority for a client with a specific diagnosis (i.e., temperature, pulse, respiratory rate, and blood pressure) and why?

2. Which of these vital signs should be reported to a team member or provider of care for a client who is one hour post-op for a **tonsillectomy (specific diagnosis or procedure)**?

3. Which assessments would be a priority for your client (i.e., BP, bradycardia, bleeding, etc.) and why?

4. Which assessment finding is a priority for monitoring your client's hydration status (i.e., I & O, edema, signs and symptoms of dehydration)?

5. Which of your clients should be assessed/triaged initially and why?

6. Which focused assessment (or system-specific assessment) would require immediate intervention following shift report?

7. Which focused assessment (or system-specific assessment) for a client with a **specific diagnosis** would require further intervention?

8. Which systems-specific assessment or reassessments would be the priority for your client and why (**i.e. GI, respiratory, cardiac, etc.**)?

9. Which steps would be most appropriate when performing a focused assessment for (i.e., gastrointestinal, respiratory, cardiac)?

10. Which of the psychosocial, spiritual, cultural and occupational assessment findings may affect the client's care (i.e., cultural—dietary, occupational—stress, etc.)?

11. What assessments are important for planning your client's care during hospitalization (i.e., food, latex, and environmental allergies)?

12. What is important to assess with your client when learning new information about a stressful treatment plan (non-verbal cues from the psychological or physical stressor)?

13. Which assessment findings indicate an older client understands how to or has the ability to manage self-care in the home environment (i.e., community resources)?

SYSTEM-SPECIFIC LABS/TESTS

1. Place options in chronological order when obtaining a **specific diagnostic test** (i.e., glucometer).

2. Which of these clinical findings would be a priority to report for a client who is post **the test** (**i.e., lab test, biopsy, cardiac cath, etc.**)?

3. Which of these clinical assessment findings would require immediate intervention to prevent a complication for a client who is experiencing **the procedure**?

4. Which of these clinical assessment findings from a **specific diagnostic test** would require further intervention?

cont'd on next page

THE QUICK APPROACH: INQUIRY QUESTIONS FOR CLASSROOM AND CLINICAL KNOWLEDGE ORGANIZED AROUND THE "SAFETY" MODEL *(cont'd)*

ANALYSIS & CONNECTED PRIORITY NURSING CONCEPT

1. Based on the information received in shift report, which client would require an immediate nursing intervention?

2. Which client should be assessed first in order to assist with time management?

3. Which signs and symptoms indicate a complication from *a specific drug, medical condition, etc.*?

4. Place in order of care delivery how you would assess/triage these four clients.

5. Which of these clinical findings indicates a change in client's condition and needs immediate intervention?

6. Which client would be a priority for the nurse to assess first following shift report?

7. Which of these changes in the client's condition requires immediate intervention?

FIRST-DO PLANS AND INTERVENTIONS

Plans

1. Which plan would be most effective for maintaining client confidentiality/privacy?

2. What plan would be most important for a client with *Diabetes Insipidus (or any condition that requires calculation of the I & O for client)*?

3. Which behavioral management techniques would be most useful in the plan for a client who is presenting with *a specific disorder* (i.e., manipulative)?

4. What plan would be highest priority for assisting a client to sleep/rest after being discharged from the hospital?

5. What plan would be the highest priority for a client with an alteration in nutritional intake (*i.e., anorexia, pica, anemia, gastroenteritis, colitis, etc.*) (i.e., adjust diet, monitor height and weight, include food preferences, etc.)?

6. What plan would be important to include when teaching a client/family member(s) about a procedure/treatment/medical condition/medication, etc. ?

Interventions

1. What is the priority nursing action for a client with a *fluid and electrolyte imbalance* (*specific concept, i.e., hypo/hypercalcemia, hypo/hyperkalemia, increase in intracranial pressure, hypothermia, etc.*)?

2. What is the priority nursing intervention for a client with a *sodium level of 128 mEq/* or *any alteration in a lab value* (i.e., serum glucose, serum potassium, etc.)?

3. What nursing intervention has the highest priority for promoting infection control for a client with a *specific disease/organism* (i.e., TB, Rubella, Clostridium difficile, Hepatitis A, etc.)?

4. When communicating with your client, what is your best response?

5. What therapeutic communication techniques were used to support your client or family and/or increase client understanding of his/her behavior?

6. What intervention(s) would be effective in assisting client with emotional and spiritual needs?

7. Which intervention(s) would be the highest priority to manage/prevent possible complications of your client's condition and/or procedure (i.e., circulatory complications, seizures, aspiration, potential neurological complications, etc.) or a client on a ventilator?

8. What would be the priority of care for a client who has been physically abused? (advocate, report, etc.)

9. What intervention was used to provide client and family with information about condition/illness, expected progression, and/or possible outcomes?

THE QUICK APPROACH: INQUIRY QUESTIONS FOR CLASSROOM AND CLINICAL KNOWLEDGE ORGANIZED AROUND THE "SAFETY" MODEL *(cont'd)*

10. What procedures did you implement in order to admit, transfer, or discharge the client?

11. What steps did you take in discontinuing or removing: IV, NG, urethral catheter, or other lines or tubes?

12. Which nursing intervention would be a priority for providing therapy for comfort and treatment of inflammation, swelling (i.e., apply heat and cold treatments, elevate limb, etc.)?

13. What are the appropriate steps in performing or assisting with a dressing change (i.e., wound, central line dressing, etc.)?

14. How can you provide the appropriate support to a client coping with life changes?

15. What is the priority of care when transcribing healthcare provider orders for a new prescription for $MgSO_4$? (*Unapproved abbreviation*)

16. Which nursing action is appropriate for proper lifting, assistive devices, etc. (*using ergonomic principles*)?

17. What nursing action would be appropriate for a client with a new order that you have limited knowledge about (i.e., *information technology such as computer, video, etc.*)?

18. What nursing action is the highest priority for handling bio-hazardous materials?

19. Which nursing action is highest priority when inserting, maintaining, or removing a peripheral intravenous line?

20. When managing the client on telemetry, which assessment finding should be reported for a client with a suspected **myocardial infarction or any condition that would alter the cardiac rhythm** (i.e., *angina, hyperkalemia, hypokalemia, overdose of digitalis, etc.*)?

21. Which intervention is the highest priority for a client with an alteration in **elimination** (i.e., **cystitis, constipation, diarrhea, etc.**)?

22. When providing care what evidence-based practice/research results did you use for providing quality care to your client?

23. What nursing action is the highest priority immediately prior to the client going to **specific surgery or procedure** in the AM? (*Answer: Check that informed consent is on the chart.*)

24. What nursing action is the highest priority immediately 2 days prior to the client going to **specific surgery or procedure**? (*Answer: Verify client comprehends and consents to care/procedures, including procedures requiring informed consent.*)

25. What nursing care would be most appropriate for a client with (*i.e.*, **anxiety, depression, dementia, eating disorders**)?

26. What is the priority of care for a client presenting with **specific clinical findings** indicating alteration in *hemodynamics tissue perfusion and hemostasis* (i.e., cerebral, cardiac, peripheral)?

27. What nursing care is a priority following a **specific surgery** and is presenting with **specific clinical assessment findings** (i.e., *thyroidectomy, tonsillectomy, GI surgery, hysterectomy, etc.*)?

FIRST-DO MEDICATIONS

1. Prior to administering the medication, which data would be most pertinent to review (i.e., vital signs, lab results, allergies, etc.)?

2. When adjusting or titrating dosage of medications, what physiological parameters did you use (i.e., giving insulin according to blood sugar levels, titrating medication to maintain a specified blood pressure, etc.)?

3. Which nursing actions will be most appropriate with medication administration (using the rights of medication administration)?

cont'd on next page

THE QUICK APPROACH: INQUIRY QUESTIONS FOR CLASSROOM AND CLINICAL KNOWLEDGE ORGANIZED AROUND THE "SAFETY" MODEL *(cont'd)*

4. During an IV infusion, what is most important to monitor and maintain (*i.e., infusion site, equipment, flushing infusion devices, checking, rates, fluid, and sites, etc.*)?

5. What is the priority intervention for your client who is receiving medication by the *intravenous route (i.e., IVP, IVPB, PCA pump, continuous infusion fluids, parenteral nutrition) or by SC, IM, intradermal or topical or in the form of eye, ear or nose drops, sprays, ointments or by inhalation (including nebulizer or metered dose inhaler)*?

6. Which calculations did you use for medication administration?

7. What regulations did you comply with when working with controlled substances (i.e., counting narcotics, wasting narcotics, etc.)?

8. What information did you share with the client/family regarding the medication regimen, treatments, and/or procedures?

9. What would be the priority of care when transcribing health care provider orders for a new prescription for $MgSO_4$?

10. What steps are most important when administering medications by the oral route or gastric tube (i.e., po, sublingual, nasogastric tube, G tube, etc.)?

11. What plan is most appropriate for preparing medication for administration (i.e., crush medications as needed and appropriate, place in appropriate administrative device, assemble equipment, etc.)?

12. What should be included in the plan to avoid when administering medications (i.e., food, fluids, and other drugs) to minimize medication interactions?

13. What clinical outcomes best determine the effect of the (*pain medication—specific medication*)?

14. What clinical findings are expected when the dopamine dosage is titrated appropriately?

15. What clinical findings are expected when the insulin is titrated according to the blood sugar levels?

16. Which assessment findings indicate a positive outcome from the albuterol (Ventolin) treatment?

17. Which assessment findings indicate positive outcomes from (*specific medications*)?

18. Which documentation indicates the nurse understands standard terminology and how to use approved abbreviations?

19. Which clinical findings indicate a therapeutic effect from *a specific drug*?

20. What is most important to monitor for a client with (i.e., central, PICC, epidural, and venous access)?

21. What plan for a client taking *warfarin (Coumadin) (or a specific medication)* would reflect care within the legal scope of practice?

22. What is the priority of care for a client prior to the nurse initiating any procedure, care, or medication administration?

23. What information is most important to include in the teaching plan for a client who has an order for (*specific medication*)?

24. What is the priority of care for a client who has a central line?

25. Which of these *medications* should the nurse question the appropriateness for a specific client?

26. Which of these *orders* should the nurse question?

27. Which of these *orders* should be verified for appropriateness/accuracy?

28. What would be the priority of care for a LPN who administered (*specific medication such as propranolol*) for a client with asthma?

THE QUICK APPROACH: INQUIRY QUESTIONS FOR CLASSROOM AND CLINICAL KNOWLEDGE ORGANIZED AROUND THE "SAFETY" MODEL *(cont'd)*

29. Which of these assessment findings require immediate intervention?

30. Which plan is priority for a client when the nurse is administering medication in order to maintain a safe and controlled environment?

PROCEDURES

1. After a specific diagnostic test (*i.e., cardiac catheterization, liver biopsy, stress test, etc.*), what clinical outcomes indicate a complication?

2. Which of these results from (*a specific diagnostic test*) indicate a complication?

3. When performing a diagnostic test (i.e., O_2 saturation, glucose monitoring, testing for occult blood, gastric pH, urine specific gravity, etc.) what are the most important interventions?

4. What nursing action would be important for the nurse to implement prior to performing a specific diagnostic test? (i.e., electrocardiogram, oxygen saturation, glucose monitoring, etc.)

5. What nursing intervention would be highest priority for a client who has (*a specific complication after a diagnostic test*) (*i.e., bleeding after a liver biopsy, bleeding after a cardiac catheterization, etc.*)

6. What nursing action would be important when obtaining *a urine specimen from a catheter* or (*i.e., wound specimen, stool, etc.*)?

7. Which information would be important to teach a client regarding *a specific treatment/procedure*?

8. Which clinical findings following a (*specific diagnostic test*) require further intervention in order to prevent complications?

9. What is important to include in the plan when assisting with an invasive procedure (*i.e., thoracentesis, bronchoscopy, etc.*)?

10. Which of these vital signs following a (*specific diagnostic test*) require further intervention?

EVALUATION OF OUTCOMES

1. What clinical findings indicate effectiveness of treatment for a client with *a specific acute or chronic diagnosis*? (*i.e., Parkinson's Disease, Multiple Sclerosis, etc.*)

2. What is important to evaluate with the client who is using a device to promote venous return such as (*i.e., anti-embolic stockings, sequential compression devices*)?

3. What plan would be appropriate for evaluating the care of a client (*i.e., evaluate care map, clinical pathway, etc.*)?

4. What documentation is most appropriate for a procedure, treatment, or medication and what is the client's response?

5. Is the medication order appropriate for your client (*i.e., appropriate for the client's condition, given by appropriate route, in appropriate dosage, etc.*)?

6. What documentation in the chart indicates an understanding of the appropriate education necessary for client and family regarding pain management?

7. Which documentation evaluates teaching performed and the level of understanding of client, family or staff?

8. Which documentation indicates the client and family have been educated about his/her rights and responsibilities?

9. Which documentation indicates that the client has given informed consent for treatment?

10. What assessment findings indicate an improvement in the client's hydration status?

cont'd on next page

THE QUICK APPROACH: INQUIRY QUESTIONS FOR CLASSROOM AND CLINICAL KNOWLEDGE ORGANIZED AROUND THE "SAFETY" MODEL *(cont'd)*

11. After initiating the plan of care, how did you evaluate the client care (i.e., multidisciplinary care plan, care map, critical pathway, etc.)?

12. Which clinical findings indicate a need to evaluate the client's weight?

13. What clinical outcomes best determine the effect of the pain medication?

14. What assessment findings indicate an improvement in the client's hydration status?

15. What clinical assessment findings indicate desired outcomes from a (*i.e., specific medication, intervention, procedure, test, etc.*)?

16. What clinical assessment findings indicate a complication from a (*i.e., specific medication, intervention, procedure, test, etc.*)?

TREND POTENTIAL COMPLICATIONS

1. Which trends and changes in client condition require further intervention?

2. Which signs and symptoms indicate complications? What is the priority intervention?

3. Which vital signs, I & O, hemodynamic readings, intracranial pressure readings, Glasgow Coma Scale number, lab values, breath sounds, etc. require further evaluation and intervention?

YOU MUST MANAGE CARE: PREVENT "RISKs"

Room Assignments, **R**ecognize limitations of staff, **R**estraint safety, **R**isk for falls, **R**ecognize cost-effective care

1. Which plan would be most appropriate to protect your client from injury (*i.e., falls, electrical hazards, malfunctioning equipment, rugs, clutter, etc.*)?

2. What is the plan for assisting the client in the performance of activities of daily living (*i.e., ambulation, reposition, hygiene, transfer to chair, eating, toileting, etc.*)?

3. What plan is most important to develop after evaluating the risk assessment profile for your client (*i.e., sensory impairment, potential for falls, level of mobility, etc.*) *and why*?

4. What plan would be most cost-effective for the nurse manager to implement on medical surgical unit?

5. Which of the clients would be most appropriate to transfer to the (i.e., medical surgical unit, orthopedic, psychiatric, etc.) unit?

6. While supervising the (i.e., UAP, LPN, RN) the nurse observes the **UAP (*palpating the abdomen of a child with Wilm's tumor*)** (*include an unsafe nursing practice*). What would be the priority nursing action?

7. What would be the priority action from the charge nurse for a LPN who administered ***propranolol or a specific medication*** for a client with ***asthma or a specific disease***?

8. What room assignment would be most appropriate for a client with TB?

9. What is the priority of care for a client with an order for restraints?

10. Which nursing action for a client with restraints on requires immediate intervention?

THE QUICK APPROACH: INQUIRY QUESTIONS FOR CLASSROOM AND CLINICAL KNOWLEDGE ORGANIZED AROUND THE "SAFETY" MODEL *(cont'd)*

Infection Control, Identification of client, Identify accuracy of orders, Informed consent, Interdisciplinary Collaboration

1. Which **assessment findings** would result in the nurse developing a plan to collaborate with *other disciplines* (i.e., physician, RT, PT, radiology, dietary, lab, etc.) while providing care to the client with a **specific diagnosis**?

2. What would be a priority plan for a client who is providing care for husband with (*i.e., Alzheimer's Disease—or a specific disease*) and is presenting with (*i.e., fatigue and weight loss—or specific assessment findings*)? *(referral)*

3. What nursing intervention would have the highest priority for promoting infection control for a client with **the specific communicable disease (i.e., TB, C. Diff, Salmonella, etc.)**?

4. Which nursing actions indicate an understanding of safe care for a client with **tuberculosis (specific disease)**?

5. What would be the priority of care when transcribing the health care provider's new order for a prescription for **MgSO₄**?

6. What is the priority of care for a client presenting with delusions who needs a medication and does not have an arm bracelet on for identification?

7. What is the priority of care for a client prior to going to surgery?

Skin breakdown, Safe equipment, Standard of Practice, Scope of Practice for delegation

1. What is the priority plan for maintaining your client's skin integrity (i.e., skin care, turn client, etc.)?

2. What plan is most appropriate when using equipment in performing **specific client care procedures and treatment**?

3. What is the appropriate nursing care for **devices and equipment** used for drainage (i.e., surgical wound drains, chest tube suction, or drainage devices, urethral catheter care, etc.)?

4. Which **level of nursing personnel** would be most appropriate to assign to a client with **specific condition/assessments**, etc. when making out assignments (i.e., LPN, VN, assistive personnel, other RNs, etc.)?

5. Which of these nursing interventions are consistent with the Standards of Practice for a client with a **specific disease**?

Know how to Document, Know how to Teach, Know Ethical Practice, Know Growth and Development

1. Which plan would be most important in meeting the special needs of the adult client who is (**? years old**) (19-64 years of age)?

2. Which plan would be most important in meeting the special needs of the adult client who is (**? years old**) (65-85 years of age) (over 85 years)?

3. What would be a plan necessary for the parents of a newborn (*i.e., education*)?

4. What information regarding healthy behaviors and health promotion / maintenance recommendations would be appropriate for (*i.e., pregnant woman, infant, post-menopausal, smoker, etc.*)?

5. What is important to include in the discharge teaching plan for a client going home after being diagnosed with a **cerebral vascular accident** (*i.e., home safety issues*)?

6. What nursing action indicates the nurse understands the code of ethics for the registered nurse?

7. Which documentation indicates client understands newly learned information?

8. Which documentation indicates an understanding of safe medication administration for a client who received (**i.e. specific medication**)?

Adapted from NCSBN, 2015. *Organized within the SAFETY Model* by I CAN Publishing, Inc., 2016

APPENDIX C

EXAMPLE OF REFLECTION QUESTIONS

Student Name _____ Clinical Instructor _____

Sec # _____ Date _____ Sat/UnSat or Grade _____

Date due to Clinical Instructor: _____

Six (6) points are possible and will be added to Rubric Grading Tool for the Concept Map
(see Chapter 4, Appendix B)

1. Connect the clinical findings (diagnostic test results) to the priority interventions (medications, treatments) for your client and provide the rationale. (2 points)

2. Based on your analysis of the concepts, what are the expected outcomes for your client? (2 points)

3. What went well today for you in clinical and why? (1 point)

4. What would you do differently if you could and why? (1 point)

URINARY CATHETERIZATION ALGORITHM

Expected Outcome: Urinary flow established through the catheter while maintaining asepsis and client comfort.

Inquiry and Reflection Questions about Insertion of a Foley Catheter

Why does this client need a Foley catheter? (Application)
Possible answers: Fluid management, incontinence, post-op renal or urinary procedures

What are potential complications for this client with a Foley catheter? (Application)
Possible answers: Urinary tract infections, skin irritations

What is important to assess in this client with a Foley catheter? (Application)
Possible answers: I & O, signs of infection, color, odor, amount of urine

What are the infection control issues for this client with a Foley catheter? (Application)
Possible answers: Sterile procedure, potential UTI from the catheter, obtaining specimens

Have you done this procedure before?

YES   NO

What went well with that procedure? (Assessing)   Name steps of procedure. (Knowledge)
Did the procedure go as planned? (Reflection)   What potential complications do you anticipate
What will you do differently next time? (Reflection)   with this client? (Analysis)
                                                        What are possible solutions to these
                                                           potential complications? (Analysis)

Clinical instructor observes the student doing the procedure.

Clinical instructor evaluates the procedure or process.

Was the student able to give individualized care with the task?

T – Techniques of communication with consideration of the individual

A – Assessment, A & P, Asepsis

S - Safety

K – Knowledge and correct implementation of the procedure/skill

YES   NO

Give positive feedback based on **TASK.**   Give feedback that the student needs improvement.

Document on evaluation form.   Give specific (TASK) feedback to the students on
                                                           their performance.
                                                        Give them specific behaviors they need to change
                                                           before performing a catheterization again.

                                                        Evaluate based on previous experience with
                                                           catheterizations.

                                                        Document on evaluation form.

APPENDIX E

THINKING STRATEGIES TO IMPROVE STUDENTS' CLINICAL REASONING

Thinking Strategies	Definitions	Faculty Strategies	Inquiry Question Examples	Reflection Question Examples
Knowledge Work	• Active use of reading, memorizing, drilling, writing, reviewing, and practicing to learn clinical vocabulary and facts.	• Set the structure and expectations required for preparation prior to clinical. • Give clear feedback on what knowledge the students need to know, i.e., drug-action of medication.	• Why does a client with heart failure have edema?	• What knowledge did I need about heart failure that I did not know? • What do I need to know before I care for a heart failure client again?
Prototype Identification	• Using a model case as a reference point for comparing and contrasting the clinical findings of your client.	• Compare students' clients to prototype in the textbooks or learned in the class room.	• How would a prototype case of heart failure present?	• Were you able to recognize how your client was different from the prototype? • What changes will you make in the care you give next time?
Hypothesizing	• Generating potential concepts based on the pathophysiology of the medical condition. • Recognizing multiple approaches to an outcome or problem.	• Have students hypothesize priority concepts, system-specific assessments, and priority interventions based on their client's admitting diagnosis(es) prior to the beginning of clinical.	• What system-specific assessments do you need to confirm or change your analysis of your concepts? • Based on your confirmed analysis of the concepts, what are your priority interventions (plan of care)?	• Was I able to identify the appropriate concepts and interventions for my client? • If not, what could I do differently?
Self-Talk	• Expressing one's thoughts to one's self	• Use self-talk, (i.e., talk aloud to the students about the what and why of your thinking).	• Talk aloud to me about how you will auscultate your client's lung sounds.	• Was I able to auscultate the lung sounds correctly; and if so, do I need to change my priority interventions?

THINKING STRATEGIES TO IMPROVE STUDENTS' CLINICAL REASONING *(cont'd)*

Thinking Strategies	Definitions	Faculty Strategies	Inquiry Question Examples	Reflection Question Examples
Schema Search	• Accessing general/specific patterns of past experiences that might apply to the current case.	• Ask the student to connect their previous experiences with the current client.	• How does this heart failure client compare to the heart failure client you took care of last week?	• Based on my experiences with heart failure clients, what patterns of care do I see?
If–Then Thinking	• Connecting ideas and consequences together in a logical sequence.	• Ask students questions about potential clinical decisions they could make and what would be the consequences of those decisions.	• If you give the medication now, what will happen? If you hold the medication, what will happen?	• Did I make the right decision about giving/holding the medication? If not, what would I do differently next time?
Compare & Contrast	• Comparing the strengths and weaknesses of competing alternatives.	• Have students identify all the interventions and select the priority intervention(s) for the client.	• What would be the most effective priority intervention(s) to help improve this client's breathing?	• Did I choose the most effective intervention to improve my client's breathing? • How did I know the intervention was effective?
Trending	• Comparing the client's clinical presentation from one observation to the next observation during the clinical day.	• Have students compare, contrast, and trend the assessments they made at the beginning of the clinical day with the assessments they make throughout the clinical day.	• What were the trends you identified in the assessments you made of your client? • Are there any changes in your assessment? • What actions do you need to take based on your assessment?	• Was I able to identify the trends and changes accurately? • Were your actions appropriate? • If yes, I knew because … • If no, I would do what differently?

ENGAGING THE LEARNER ACTIVITIES

STUDENT-CENTERED LEARNING ACTIVITIES
LINKED TO PROFESSIONAL AND NCLEX® STANDARDS

Resources Needed for Activity	*The Eight-Step Approach for Teaching Clinical Nursing* (Zager, Manning & Herman, 2017)	*The Eight-Step Approach for Student Clinical Success* (Zager, Manning & Herman, 2017)
Standards	**Faculty Instructions**	**Student Instructions**
Physiological integrity; Reduction of Risk Recognize trends and changes in VS, client condition and intervene appropriately; Recognize and prevent signs and symptoms of complications and intervene appropriately.	**Clinical Reasoning: Thinking Strategies** (Refer to Appendix E) Discuss the examples given for If–Then Thinking, Compare and Contrast and Trending. *Have students work in pairs.* 1. Describe examples of the thinking strategies used in their clinical decisions made during the clinical day (*assist students in "thinking outside the box" for their examples*): a. "If–Then Thinking." b. "Compare and Contrast." c. "Trending."	**Clinical Reasoning: Thinking Strategies** (Refer to Use Thinking Strategies to Develop Clinical Reasoning at the end of Chapter 3) 1. Based on your clinical day: a. Give an example of how you used "If–Then Thinking" in your clinical decision-making. b. Give an example of how you used "Compare and Contrast" for your clinical decision-making. c. Give an example how you used "Trending" for your clinical decision-making.
Physiological integrity; Reduction of Risk Educate and evaluate accuracy of a treatment order and response to procedures and treatments; Verify appropriateness of an order.	**Clinical Reasoning: Procedures** (Refer to Appendix D and refer students to the Procedure Template at the end of Chapter 3 in *The Eight-Step Approach for Student Clinical Success*) 2. Write different procedures (*choose procedures students know*) on index cards and have pairs of students select a card. Instruct them to answer the questions on the Procedure Template. a. Each pair of students reports their answers to the questions to the group. b. Ask the students: What are the similarities and differences to the answers for different procedures? c. Emphasize to the students that the questions they should ask themselves are the same regardless of the procedure because they are based on standards of practice.	**Clinical Reasoning: Procedures** (Refer to Urinary Catheterization Algorithm and the Procedure Template at the end of Chapter 3) 2. Work in pairs and answer the questions on the Procedure Template. a. Report your answers to the group. b. Are their similarities in your fellow students answers about their procedures and yours? c. What are the differences? d. How can you apply these questions to other procedures?

The Concept Map

IN THIS CHAPTER YOU WILL LEARN HOW TO:

➡ Discuss the advantages of a concept map compared to traditional clinical paperwork

➡ Instruct students to create and use a concept map

◊ Step 1– Begin with the admitting diagnoses

◊ Step 2 – Generate (hypothesize) possible concepts

◊ Step 3 – Determine relationships among the concepts

◊ Step 4 – Add system-specific assessment findings

◊ Step 5 – Determine expected outcomes and evaluation criteria

◊ Step 6 – Determine the priority interventions

◊ Step 7 – Evaluate and make clinical judgments about the plan of care

◊ Step 8 – Document care given and client response

➡ Putting the concept map into clinical practice

The concept map provides an excellent tool for clinical faculty to help students develop clinical reasoning skills (Daley, Morgan, & Black, 2016). It is a strategy to externalize thinking, layer levels of clinical reasoning, and promote understanding of interrelationships. It is very typical for novices to focus on one particular assessment, concept, or intervention without an understanding of the complexity and interrelationships of the care needed for the client. The concept map helps students see the full scope of the client situation and assists you to see what the student is thinking about their plan of care. The chart compares the advantages of using the concept map compared to the traditional clinical paperwork in helping the students develop clinical reasoning.

**ADVANTAGES OF THE CONCEPT MAP
COMPARED TO TRADITIONAL CLINICAL PAPERWORK**

Concept Map	Traditional Clinical Paperwork
Visual picture of the interrelationships among the problems/concepts	Concepts seen in isolation
Systems approach	Linear approach
Outcome thinking	Problem thinking
Focuses on priorities of care	Focuses on medical/disease
Clinical decision-making	Task oriented
Less time to grade	Time consuming to grade
Total pages 1–2	Depends on number of concepts and can go on and on …

Adapted from Pesut & Herman, 1999

The concept map is considered the standard format for teaching students clinical reasoning (Daley, Morgan, & Black, 2016). It is imperative that clinical instructors are knowledgeable about how to guide students in constructing a concept map. We will guide you on a step-by-step approach to creating and using the concept map. The concept map can seem overwhelming when you first look at it, but when approaching it sequentially, it is easy to master for you and your students.

Teaching point: We recommend that students complete their hypothesized concept map in pencil prior to their assessment of the client. Once the students have completed their assignment, have them make any changes to their initial concept map in different color ink/pencil so you can see what changes they have made based on their assessment findings. It is important to emphasize to the students that changes they make are not wrong, but are actually an indication of their ability to clinical reason based on the ongoing changes in their client and the required care needed. The concept map should be a working document during the day that reflects the plan of care based on the client's priority needs.

HOW TO INSTRUCT STUDENTS TO CONSTRUCT AND USE A CONCEPT MAP

Students begin clinical by receiving their client assignment with the medical diagnoses. The **SAFETY Model** (See Chapter 8)/nursing process guides the steps in the development of the concept map.

STEP 1: Begin with the Admitting Diagnoses

Place the admitting medical diagnoses/client situation in the middle of the paper with any client history that would impact the current admission.

Med DX: i.e., heart failure (HF)

Pertinent History/Information (i.e., history of Chronic Renal Disease & non-compliance with low-sodium diet, etc.)

Client Age: _____

HT_____WT_____

Allergies:_____

STEP 2: Generate (Hypothesize) Possible Concepts

Have the students generate (hypothesize) possible concepts that are pathophysiologically associated with the medical diagnoses. Draw a line from the middle circle to each of the hypothesized concepts.

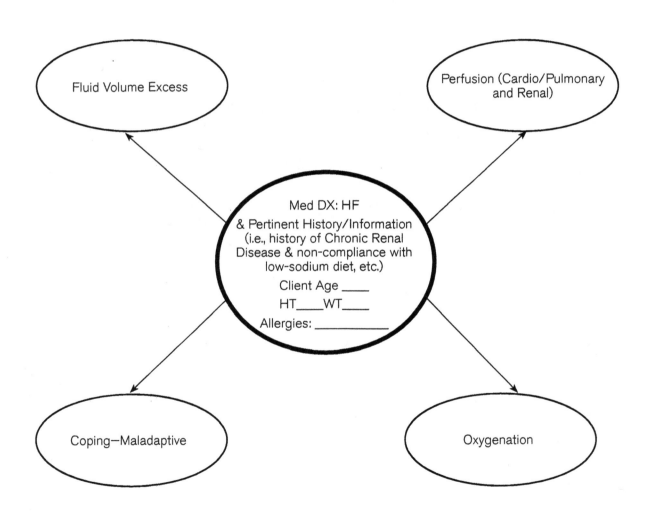

STEP 3: Determine Relationships Among the Concepts

Here is what you would say to your students to help them determine the relationships among the concepts: *"Is there any pathophysiological reason why these two concepts might be related to each other?"* (Refer to Manning & Zager, 2014).

a. *"Is there any pathophysiological reason why perfusion would be related to excess fluid volume?"*

b. In this example, the answer is yes, so draw a line connecting the two concepts.

c. Working systematically around the concept map, you will ask yourself, *"Is perfusion related to the other concepts included on the map?"*

d. Now ask, *"Is there any pathophysiological reason why perfusion is related to oxygenation?"*

e. The answer is yes. Draw a line between the two concepts.

f. Next question, *"Is there any pathophysiological reason why excess fluid volume is related to oxygenation?"*

g. The answer is yes. Draw a line between the two concepts.

h. Next, *"Is there any pathophysiological or logical reason why maladaptive coping is related to fluid volume excess?"*

i. The answer is yes. Draw a line between the two concepts.

j. Finally, *"Is there any pathophysiological reason why maladaptive coping is related to perfusion and/or oxygenation?"*

k. The answer is yes. Both perfusion and oxygenation are indirectly impacted by maladaptive coping (i.e., failure to follow a low-sodium diet) that contributes to fluid volume excess.

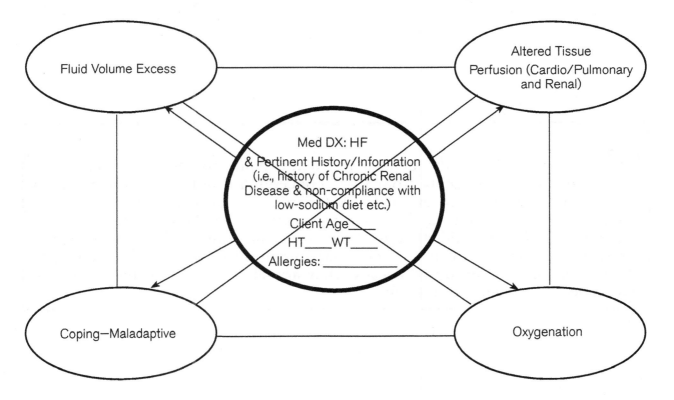

As you can see, all of these concepts are interrelated.

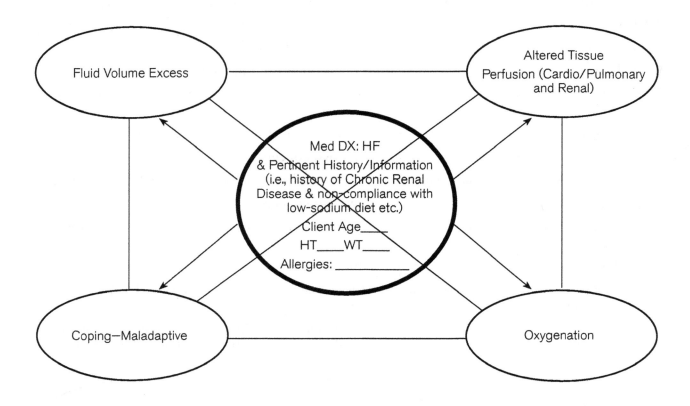

✏️ *Teaching point*: As the clinical instructor, guide the students to identify the priority client concepts from what concepts are not a priority. Students often want to include anxiety and risk for infection on every client's concept map. Yes, it is important for the students to assess for anxiety and take steps to prevent infection, but add these to the concept map only if the system-specific assessments support it or it is a potential complication for specific client (i.e., client is immunocompromised because they are taking corticoid steroids and/or have a decreased white count, etc.).

STEP 4: Add System-Specific Assessment Findings

After the student has completed their assessment of the client, add the system-specific assessment findings to the concept map. For example:

System-Specific Assessments for Fluid Volume Excess:

Weight 124 lbs. – 4 lb. gain/24 hours

SOB with activity

Lungs clear bilaterally

2+ pitting edema bilaterally in lower legs

Each client's concept chosen by the student will have system-specific assessments that confirm that the hypothesized concepts are correct. It is important that the student compare their system-specific assessment findings with the system-specific assessments that define the concept (Manning & Zager, 2014). Today's new graduate nurse must be able to not only identify the current clinical findings but be able to anticipate potential complications that could occur in the future. These potential complications may be associated with the pathophysiological changes that could occur related to the client's medical diagnosis.

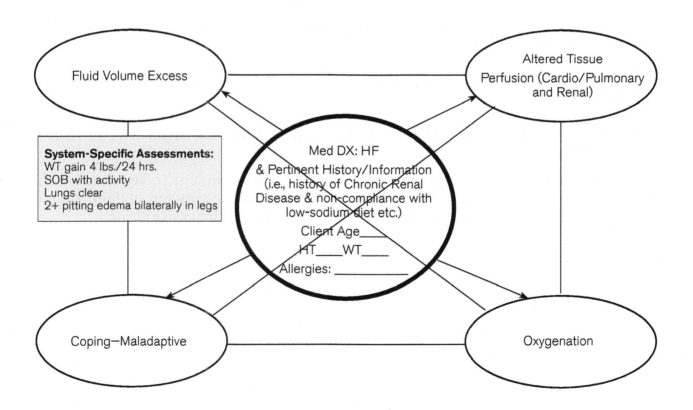

In the example on page 49, the lungs are clear bilaterally. This does not mean the student would stop assessing for adventitious lungs sounds with a client with heart failure who has fluid volume excess. The monitoring, comparing, contrasting, and trending of the clinical assessment findings leads to early identification and/or prevention of potential complications. You are teaching an expected and essential competency required of a new graduate nurse that directly impacts the quality and safety care of the client.

✏️ *Teaching point*: After reviewing the system-specific assessment findings with the students, you want to evaluate if they have identified the priority clinical assessment findings for the concept of Fluid Volume Excess. If they, for example, left out daily weight as a priority clinical assessment finding, review with them why monitoring daily weight is the best method of determining fluid status in a client (Manning & Zager, 2014).

Assuming in this case they have included the priority clinical assessment findings, ask the following inquiry questions:

1. *"What clinical findings indicate that your client may have fluid volume excess?"*

2. *"I notice you stated the client gained 4 lbs."* Is this a weight gain over the past week or in the past 24 hours?

Let's assume for teaching purposes, the student says they do not know. Your next question would be:

3. *"Why would this be important to know if your client gained or lost weight in the past 24 hours?"*

Using these inquiry questions, you are guiding your student to see that a 4 lb. weight gain in 24 hours is a significant clinical finding for the concept of fluid volume excess. This process is repeated for all of the concepts on the concept map.

STEP 5: Determine Expected Outcomes and Evaluation Criteria

Determining expected outcomes and evaluation criteria are very difficult for students because they have little clinical experience. They have great difficulty with outcome-focused thinking because it requires a high level of clinical reasoning (Pesut & Herman, 1999). Here is an easy way to teach students how to develop outcomes. Transform the concept into a positive term. For example, let's take the concept "fluid volume excess" and ask, "What is the desired outcome for a client with fluid volume excess?" The answer is "Fluid Volume Balance" … voila the **OUTCOME!**

The next step is to determine if the desired outcome was met and if so, how do you know it was met? You develop evaluation criteria using the same process you used for the system-specific assessments and transform them into desired outcomes. For example, one of the assessments for excess fluid volume is "weight gain of 4 pounds since yesterday." The desired outcome can be measured by the evaluation criterion of "weight gain < 2 lbs. per day."

The following table illustrates the outcome and evaluation criteria development process for all of the concepts used in this example.

DETERMINE OUTCOMES AND EVALUATION CRITERIA TABLE

Concepts	System-Specific Assessments	Outcome	Outcome Criteria
Fluid Volume Excess	• Weight gain of 4 lbs from yesterday • Lungs clear • SOB with activity • 2+ pitting edema bilaterally lower peripheral extremities	Fluid Volume Balance	• Wt gain < 2 lbs/day • Lungs clear • No SOB • No edema bilaterally
Oxygenation	• c/o of SOB • c/o of anxiety • Respirations 23/minute • O_2 Sat 91%	Adequate Oxygenation	• No SOB • No c/o of anxiety • Respirations 16–20/min • O_2 Sat > 95%
Perfusion–Cardiac/ Peripheral/Renal	• Capillary refill > 3 sec • Pulses + 1 • Heart rate 88 bpm • Urine 50mL/hr	Adequate Tissue Perfusion	• Capillary refill < 3 sec • Pulses +2 • HR 60–100 bpm • Urine > 30mL/hr
Coping– Maladaptive	• Spouse recently died • Buying processed prepared food for meals • High intake of salt due to processed prepared food • No interest in preparing own meals	Coping–Adaptive	• Met with nutritionist • Connected with grief support group • Able to identify foods with high Na^+ content • Demonstrates interest in preparing own meals

(Manning & Zager, 2014)

STEP 6: Determine Priority Interventions

Determining the priority interventions for the client is the next step. The nursing interventions *italicized* in the chart on page 53 are priority because they help achieve more than one client outcome. The other interventions are distinct to that particular concept and outcome.

When a student sees all of the interventions on a concept map, the student is able to determine which interventions will be most effective for the most outcomes. This exercise helps the students see the client as a whole (system thinking) versus looking at each client's concepts and outcome separately (linear thinking). Using the same client, the table illustrates this process with the four concepts used.

Teaching Point: Clinical instructors will want to use inquiry and reflection questions to help the students understand why a particular intervention would help achieve the outcome. For example, the assessment finding of 3+ pitting edema bilaterally in the lower peripheral extremities indicates to the student the need for further interventions.

1. *"What intervention would help decrease peripheral edema?"* You hope this question will lead the students to the intervention of positioning.

2. *"What position would best help the client decrease edema?"* This question would guide the student to the intervention of elevating the legs to the level of the heart.

3. As the student's clinical reasoning develops during the semester, increase the complexity of the inquiry questions. For example, *"Which of the medications is the client taking that will assist in achieving the expected outcomes?"*

DEVELOPING OUTCOMES AND EVALUATION CRITERIA WITH INTERVENTIONS

The italicized interventions are priority because they help achieve more than one client outcome.

Concepts	System-Specific Assessments	Outcome	Outcome Criteria	Priority Interventions
Fluid Volume Excess	• Weight gain of 4 lbs from yesterday • Lungs clear • SOB with activity • 2+ pitting edema bilaterally lower peripheral extremities	Fluid Volume Balance	• Wt gain < 2 lbs/day • Lungs clear • No SOB • No edema bilaterally	• Weigh daily, compare & trend • Assess I & O q 8 hrs. • *Assess lung sounds* • *Cough and deep breathe q 4 hrs.* • *Incentive spirometer every hour while awake* • *Semi-Fowler's position with legs elevated at heart level* • *Assess SOB q 4 hrs.* • *Assess edema q 4 hrs.*
Oxygenation	• c/o of SOB • c/o of anxiety • Respirations 23/minute • O_2 Sat 91% with 2L O_2/Nasal cannula • Lungs clear bilaterally	Adequate Oxygenation	• No SOB • Lungs clear • Respirations 16–20/min • O_2 Sat > 95%	• Assess SOB • Assess for restlessness • Assess RR and O_2 sat • Administer O_2 as ordered • *Assess lung sounds* • *Cough and deep breathe q 4 hrs.* • *Incentive spirometer every hour while awake* • *Semi-Fowler's position*
Perfusion—Cardiac/Peripheral/Renal	• Capillary refill > 3 sec • Pulses +1 • Heart rate 88 bpm • Urine 50 mL/hr	Adequate Perfusion—Cardiac/Peripheral/Renal	• Capillary refill < 3 sec • Pulses +2 bilaterally • Skin warm and dry • Color pink • HR 60–100 bpm • Urine > 30 mL/hr	• Assess capillary refill q 4 hrs. • Assess HR, pulses bilaterally, color & skin temp q 4 hrs. • *Position with legs at heart level* • *HOB Semi-Fowler's position* • Report urine output < 30 mL/hr or trending ↓
Coping—Maladaptive	• Spouse recently died • Buying processed prepared food for meals • No interest in preparing own meals • High intake of salt due to processed prepared food	Coping—Adaptive	• Collaborative—met with nutritionist • Connected with grief support group • Demonstrates an interest in preparing own meals • Able to identify sources of high Na^+ foods	• Consult to dietary • Assist client in selecting low sodium food from the menu • Consult to grief support group or spiritual advisor

(Manning & Zager, 2014)

STEP 7: Evaluate Outcomes and Make Clinical Judgments About the Plan of Care

The next step is to determine if outcomes have been achieved. This is not a yes or no answer, but a process of comparing the evaluation criteria to the client's current system-specific assessments. There are three clinical judgments that are possible.

✦ Outcome met

✦ Outcome partially met

✦ Outcome not met

Now that a decision about outcome achievement has been made, the clinical instructor needs to help the students decide what the plan of care will be. What are their nursing responsibilities? This is clinical judgment. Clinical judgment uses a series of reflective questions and decisions to plan future client care as indicated in the questions below.

OUTCOME NOT MET

1. Did the client's situation change (i.e., developed adventitious lung sounds)?
   a. If yes, revise plan of care to correspond to the new client condition.
   b. If no, go on to the next question.

2. Did the interventions fail to be effective?
   a. If yes, revise the interventions.
   b. If no, go on to the next question.

3. Did I evaluate too soon or is more time needed for the interventions to be effective?
   a. If yes, continue the current care and continue to evaluate.
   b. If no, go to next question.

4. Were the conclusions drawn from the system-specific assessment findings accurate?
   a. If yes, continue the current plan of care and continue to evaluate.
   b. If no, re-analyze the system-specific assessment findings to determine correct client concept and outcome, and revise the plan of care.

OUTCOME PARTIALLY ACHIEVED

If the outcome was partially achieved, then the student would use similar reflection questions.

1. Is more time needed for the interventions to be effective?
   a. If yes, continue the current plan of care and continue to evaluate.
   b. If no, go to next question.
2. Are changes needed in the interventions to achieve the outcome?
   a. If yes, make the changes (i.e., increase the frequency of the interventions or add new interventions, etc.).
   b. If no, continue plan of care and ongoing evaluation.

OUTCOME ACHIEVED

1. Is the problem likely to recur without nursing interventions?
   a. If no, discontinue plan of care.
   b. If yes, go to next question.
2. Does the concept require the same level of intervention or vigilance?
   a. If yes, continue plan of care.
   b. If no, revise plan of care to meet current client needs.

It is common for the student to say, "The client does not have this concept as a problem because they have no system-specific assessments to confirm the concept, so I need to take it off the concept map."

For example, it is very important that the student understand there is high risk of recurrence of fluid volume excess in a client with heart failure (HF) and renal failure. *It would not be safe practice to quit monitoring for the clinical findings of fluid volume excess even if the client's weight is stable and the lungs are clear. The problem is likely to recur due to the pathophysiological changes that occur with heart failure.* The prudent nurse will monitor for potential complications. Therefore, fluid volume excess would remain on the concept map. Here are two examples of inquiry questions to help guide the students in this judgment process:

1. *"Your client has HF with renal failure; what is the risk that fluid volume excess may recur?"*
2. *"What would you want to continue to monitor to prevent complications?"*

STEP 8:   Document Care Given and Client Response

After making a clinical judgment, students will need to document their conclusions in the medical record. The concept map is a useful guide for students while they document. It is important that documentation contain the following information:

+ Client's system-specific assessments

+ Client's response to priority interventions

+ Progress toward the expected outcomes

+ Any changes in the plan of care

The concept map and the student's clinical notes should provide all of the information the student needs to document accurately.

PUT THE CONCEPT MAP INTO CLINICAL PRACTICE

The development of the concept map begins when students receive their clinical assignments. If a student is not able to assess the assigned client, they can begin the concept map using a prototype case (see Chapter 3). The concept map may change after the student actually assesses their client (see Teaching Point on page 44).

The table **Putting the Concept Map into Clinical Practice** describes how the clinical instructor can help the student apply the concept map.

Interaction between the clinical instructor and the student is similar as the student works through each of the remaining steps 3 through 7 in constructing the concept map.

The concept map is an established best practice for teaching students clinical reasoning (Daley, Morgan, & Black, 2016). Using the concept map does require practice and repetition on both the part of the clinical instructor and the students. When the concept map is used in each clinical experience through a curriculum, the concept map becomes an internalized part of the students' thinking. The students are able to transition from the written concept map to oral presentations of the concept map in their last semesters of school. Systematic thinking, once illustrated through a written concept map, becomes a clinical reasoning habit students will use in their clinical practice.

PUTTING THE CONCEPT MAP INTO CLINICAL PRACTICE

Student Responsibility	Clinical Instructor Responsibility	Teaching Points
1. Hypothesize the concepts around the assigned client's medical diagnosis(es)and bring your concept map to clinical.	• Review the hypothesized concept map at the beginning of clinical based on the prototype client. Note: you will need to allow time for the students to do this if they receive their assignment at the beginning of clinical instead of the day before. (With practice, students can do this in 15 minutes!) • Have students complete the pathophysiology, lab, and AIDES sheet while they are learning (see Chapter 3).	• Does the concept map reflect the prototype client for this medical diagnosis(es)? If so, go to number 3 under Student Responsibility. • *Remember that the concept map will not have individualized care at this point.* • *If the concept map does not reflect the priority concepts, then this is a teaching opportunity to guide the student. Go to number 2 under Student Responsibility.*
2. If your hypothesized concepts are incorrect after speaking with your clinical instructor, then edit or add to the concept map. *Hint: Initially use a pencil to complete concept map. Use different color pencil/ink for different concepts. DO NOT ERASE; just put an X through the revision or change colors, so you can see the CHANGE in THINKING and LEARN from this. Do not start over! This reflects your ability to clinically reason.*	• Guide the students to include concepts that would be part of the prototype client. • After the assessment, the students can cross through what was not priority and add what they assessed. • Instruct the students NOT to erase and start over. Using this process, you can see the change in the students' thinking and ability to clinically reason.	• *(Expectation of what the student should have done will be based on the level of student in clinical.)* • It is important to remind students that what they did the night before was not a waste of time. The work provides a basis for their initial system specific assessments of their client. • Then the student must organize the assessment data to determine if the selected concepts are correct or if there are additional concepts that are a priority to meet the needs of the client.
3. Assess your client and revise concept map as appropriate.	• Re-evaluate the concept map as the student makes changes. • *(This may be done orally during the clinical day, depending on the level of the student's clinical development.)*	• If after the initial assessment of the client, the student needs to make revisions in the concept map, it is the responsibility of the clinical instructor to help the student realize this is part of the process.

For your reference, at the end of this chapter is an **Example of Adult Health Concept Map** (Appendix A) and a **Rubric Grading Tool for the Adult Health Concept Map Example** (Appendix B). A blank **Adult Health Concept Map Tool** can be found in Appendix C. The rubric can be adjusted based on the course, the level of the course. and points assigned. For example, in children and family, it would be important to include developmental levels expected for the client's age according to Piaget and Erickson and to evaluate if the student understands how to correctly calculate hourly fluid requirements. Maternal and newborn would need to include evaluation of assessment of the mother, fetus, and newborn during and post-delivery.

Additional clinical forms that we have found helpful and can be adapted to your needs are: **AIDES Medication Information Tool** (Appendix D), **Reflection Questions Example** (Appendix E), **History and Pathophysiology Information Tool** (Appendix F), **Health History and System-Specific Assessment Tool** (Appendix G), and **Lab, Diagnostic Tests, and Procedure Recording Tool** (Appendix H). Concept Map Tools for other courses—**Nursing Foundations/Fundamentals** (Appendix I), **Children and Families** (Appendix J), **Maternal and Newborn** (Appendix K), and **Mental Health** (Appendix L)—can also be found at the end of the chapter.

The advantage of using the same structure for the concept maps and the rubrics is the novice student does not have to learn what each clinical instructor wants. The structure remains the same with a few differences to reflect the clinical specialty area. Using the same structure is not only beneficial to the students but it decreases the need for each faculty member in different courses to create their own clinical forms.

Teaching Point: The example provided has four concepts. Obviously, the number of concepts will vary depending on the individual client. It will also depend on the clinical development of the student. In the beginning Foundations Course, it may be appropriate to have the student only identify one concept as they are learning the process. By the senior year, students should identify all priority concepts for the client. The reality is a very acutely ill complex client may have 5 to 7 priority concepts. It is a faculty decision to decide how many concepts the student will be required to include on the concept map. We recommend 2 priority concepts in the foundations/fundamentals, obstetrics, children and family and mental health courses. At the senior level, Adult Health and Capstone courses, we recommend the students identify 3 to 4 priority concepts based on the client's needs. It is critical that students can identify the priority concepts.

EXAMPLE OF ADULT HEALTH CONCEPT MAP

Name _____ Sec # _____ Date _____ Grade _____

Clinical Faculty _____

Medical DX:
Heart Failure
History of chronic renal & non-compliance with low-sodium diet
Client Age: 68   HT: 5'8"
WT: 184 lbs.
Allergies: NKA

Concept: Perfusion Cardiac/Peripheral/Renal
Outcome: Adequate Perfusion Cardiac/Peripheral/Renal

System-Specific Assessments	Priority Interventions	Outcome Criteria
Cap refill >3 sec	Assess capillary refill q 4 hrs	Capillary refill <3 sec
Pulses +1 bilaterally	Assess HR, pulses bilaterally, color & skin temp q 4 hrs	Pulses +2 bilaterally, HR 60 – 100 bpm; HR & RR return to client's baseline within 3 min
HR-88 bpm	HOB *at Semi-Fowler's position with legs at heart level*	Skin warm and dry, color pink
Urine 50 mL/hr	Report urine <30mL/ hr trending ↓	Urine output > 30 mL/hr

Meds R/T to Concept: Digoxin
Labs R/T to Concept: Digoxin level, BUN/Creat
Equipment R/T to Concept: N/A
Client/Family Teaching R/T to Concept: Teach client how to position with lying, sitting or standing to avoid constriction of blood flow & how to monitor HR & RR before & after activity.

Concept: Oxygenation
Outcome: Adequate Oxygenation

System-Specific Assessments	Priority Interventions	Outcome Criteria
c/o of SOB	HOB ↑ semi-Fowler's	No c/o of SOB
R-23/min	C & DB q 4 hrs	RR–16 to 20/min
Lungs clear bilaterally	Incentive spirometer q 1 hr while awake	Lungs clear bilaterally
O_2 Sat 91%	Assess lungs sounds, RR & O_2 Sat q 4 hrs. & PRN & before & after activity	O_2 Sat > 95%
c/o of anxiety	O_2 /Nasal cannula /order	

Meds R/T to Concept:
Labs R/T to Concept: ABGs
Equipment R/T to Concept: O_2 sat monitor, O_2, nasal cannula, incentive spirometer
Client/Family Teaching R/T to Concept: Instruct how positioning with HOB↑ expands lung capacity.

Concept: Fluid Volume Excess
Outcome: Fluid Volume Balance

System-Specific Assessments	Priority Interventions	Outcome Criteria
Wt. 124lbs – 4 lb gain/24 hrs	I & O q 8 hrs. Weigh daily, compare & trend	Wt. gain <2lbs/day
SOB with activity	↑ legs when sitting/lying (at level of heart)	No c/o of SOB
Lungs clear bilaterally	Incentive spirometer q 1 hr while awake	Lungs clear bilaterally
2+ pitting edema bilaterally in lower legs	Assess lungs sounds, RR, SOB & O_2 Sat q 4 hrs. & PRN, trend	No edema bilaterally

Meds R/T to Concept: Furosemide
Labs R/T to Concept: Electrolytes, particularly K^+, Na^+ level, BUN/Creat
Equipment R/T to Concept: scales
Client/Family Teaching R/T to Concept: Dietary consult related to selecting low-sodium foods

Concept: Coping—Maladaptive
Outcome: Coping—Adaptive

System-Specific Assessments	Priority Interventions	Outcome Criteria
Spouse recently died	Consult to dietary	Met with dietician
Buying processed food for meals	Assist client in selecting low-sodium food from the menu	Connected with grief support group or spiritual adviser
High intake of Na^+ due to processed foods	Consult to grief support group	Able to identify foods with low Na^+ content from list
No interest in preparing own meals		Able to plan menu with low-Na^+ foods

Meds R/T to Concept:
Labs R/T to Concept:
Equipment R/T to Concept:
Client/Family Teaching R/T to Concept: Dietary consult related to selecting low-Na^+ foods, grief support and group or spiritual advisor to assist with coping

To be completed and reviewed the day of clinical by: Clinical Instructor signature: _____ Date _____

cont'd on next page

APPENDIX A
Chapter 4

EXAMPLE OF ADULT HEALTH CONCEPT MAP   PAGE 2

Name _____

Evaluation of Outcome Criteria: Perfusion
- HR ↑ 98 bpm with activity, returns to resting pulse < 3 min
- Cap refill remains > 3min
- Pulses remain 1+ bilaterally
- Urine output 320 mL/8 hrs. = > 40 mL/hr

Rationale for Interventions: Urine output > 30 mL/hr indicates adequate perfusion to the kidneys. Increase in HR & RR that does not return to client's normal within 3 min indicates an increase workload on the heart with resulting decrease in oxygen provided to vital organs.

Client response to interventions: Client positioned in bed with HOB elevated and legs elevated at heart level when lying. Having difficulty prioritizing activity so HR & RR return to baseline within 3 min.

Clinical Judgment Was overall outcome met: Yes _____   Partially __x__   Not at all _____
Rationale: Explain your decision. What would you do differently? Progress is being made but because of disease processes of HF, will continually need to monitor activities and pace with rest periods as client tolerates. Teach client to pace activities. Continue plan of care.

Evaluation of Outcome Criteria: Oxygenation
- Client states SOB is better with activity
- RR decreased from 23 to 20/min
- Lungs remain clear bilaterally
- O₂ sat 94% on 2L O₂ via NC

Rationale for Interventions: Elevation of HOB allows chest expansion, promotes oxygenation. Incentive spirometer helps client take long deep breaths, O₂/NC has increased O₂ sat, need to continue to monitor O₂ sat.

Client response to interventions: Client stated ↓SOB and was able to breathe easier with the O₂ and the HOB elevated.

Clinical Judgment Was overall outcome met: Yes _____   Partially __x__   Not at all _____
Rationale: Explain your decision. What would you do differently? Client made significant improvement as indicated by decrease RR and increased O₂ sat, but needs to continue plan of care until able to keep O₂ Sat > 95% on 2 L O₂/NC.

Evaluation of Outcome Criteria: Fluid Balance
- No weight gain in 24 hrs.
- Decreased SOB with activity
- Edema remains at 2+ bilaterally
- Lungs remain clear bilaterally

Rationale for Interventions: Monitor fluid balance with daily weights and I & O q 8 hrs because excess fluid volume increases the workload on the heart.

Client response to interventions: Client verbalizing understanding of how increased Na⁺ content in the diet contributes to excess fluid that makes it difficult to breathe. Keeping legs elevated at heart level when in bed.

Clinical Judgment Was overall outcome met: Yes _____   Partially __x__   Not at all _____
Rationale: Explain your decision. What would you do differently? Client making progress but will need to continue the plan of care. Will recommend a dietary consult to help with teaching about low Na⁺ diets and a physical therapy consult to help teach client exercises to help promote venous circulation and decrease edema in lower legs.

Priority Lab/Procedures	Results/Interpretations	Nursing Indications (Pre & Post)
• Electrolytes, Na⁺ & K⁺ • BUN/Creat	• Na⁺–138 mEq/L K⁺–3.2 mEq/L • BUN 19/Creat 1.9	• Notify healthcare provider prior to giving furosemide because of low K⁺ • Continue to monitor because of HF and receiving ace inhibitor

RUBRIC GRADING TOOL FOR ADULT HEALTH CONCEPT MAP EXAMPLE

Student Name _____ Faculty _____ Date _____

Directions: Complete one **Concept Map** each week. You will get a Pass/Fail. One of the written concept maps will be graded and one will be presented orally to your clinical instructor on designated weeks. The average of the two will be 5% of your application grade. You will receive your assigned client and primary medical diagnosis(es) when you arrive for clinical, listen to report, do your assessment and then do the first page of the concept map. The concept map is a working tool, so **make appropriate changes/additions throughout the day as the clinical situation dictates. Use a different color ink or pencil to make your changes in the concept map.** Complete the first page of your concept map by the end of clinical for your clinical instructor to review and sign. The final review will be completed when all components of the concept map, AIDES sheets and reflection page are turned in/emailed to your faculty. SBAR will be given as directed or per unit protolcol.

CONCEPT MAP COMPONENTS WITH CRITERIA FOR GRADING	POINTS	CONCEPT MAP COMPONENTS WITH CRITERIA FOR GRADING	POINTS
1. Identify **3 overall outcomes and their relevant Concept label** based on medical diagnosis & clinical condition. *3 pts for each of 3 appropriate priority concepts x 3 = 9)*	___ /9 ___ P/F	8. On page 2, **evaluate the client's response** to each intervention & progress toward desired outcomes. *3 pts for accurate evaluation of outcome criteria and interventions for each overall outcome x 3 = 9*	___ /9 ___ P/F
2. Indicate client findings for focused **(system-specific) assessments for each of the 3 concepts. All key assessments included—minimum of 3 each.** *3 pts for each concept's assessment findings (3 x 3 = 9)*	___ /9 ___ P/F	9. **State if overall outcomes were met. Provide & explain a clinical decision about each outcome based on your evaluation** (i.e., continue, modify, D/C). *3 pts for each overall outcome clinical decision (3 x 3 = 9)*	___ /9 ___ P/F
3. Identify **specific measurable outcomes for concepts. All outcome criteria incl. to fully address each overall outcome—minimum of 2 each.** *4 pts for the specific outcome criteria per overall outcome (3 x 4 = 12)*	___ /12 ___ P/F	10. On page 2, **interpret priority lab/diagnostic values** related to the client's current clinical condition with **nursing indications/care.**	___ /6 ___ P/F
4. Identify at least **4 priority interventions that will help achieve outcomes: Include at least 2 action interventions** (i.e., cough & deep breathe q 2 hrs.) **& 2 priority assessments** for client's condition/response (i.e., monitor VS q 4 hrs. & compare to previous findings). *(3 x 4 = 12)*	___ /12 ___ P/F	11. On 3 AIDES medication sheets, **describe 3 medications & identify** nursing indications & desired outcome for the medications. *3 points for each medication*	___ /9 ___ P/F
5. Use **lines to show relationships** between concepts (i.e., there is a pathophysiological connection between the two concepts). Use different colored pencils/pens for each concept to draw the lines to make the relationships clearer. *Points based on relationships being valid.*	___ /4 ___ P/F	12. Complete the History and Pathophysiology Information on the form as directed. Turn in with the concept map.	___ /3 ___ P/F
6. On page 1, **indicate appropriate medications and diagnostic results pertinent to each concept.**	___ /4 ___ P/F	13. **Critical Thinking/Reflection Questions** are answered completely & clearly with appropriate detail. Answers reflect a complete understanding of the client situation.	___ /6 ___ P/F
7. On page 1, **indicate appropriate safety/equipment risks/ precautions** (fall, seizures, infection control, etc.) and **family involvement/teaching needs for each concept.**	___ /4 ___ P/F	14. Correctly prepare and give the SBAR report to clinical instructor prior to reporting of to the assigned RN	___ /4 ___ P/F
TOTAL POINTS POSSIBLE	100	**TOTAL POINTS RECEIVED**	

APPENDIX C

Chapter 4

ADULT HEALTH CONCEPT MAP TOOL

Name _____ Clinical Instructor _____ Sec # _____ Date _____ Grade _____

Medical DX:
History:
Client Age:
HT: WT:
Allergies:

Top-left concept box

Concept:		
Outcome:		
System-Specific Assessments	Priority Interventions	Outcome Criteria

Meds R/T to Concept:
Labs R/T to Concept:
Equipment R/T to Concept:
Client/Family Teaching R/T to Concept:

Top-right concept box

Concept:		
Outcome:		
System-Specific Assessments	Priority Interventions	Outcome Criteria

Meds R/T to Concept:
Labs R/T to Concept:
Equipment R/T to Concept:
Client/Family Teaching R/T to Concept:

Bottom-left concept box

Concept:		
Outcome:		
System-Specific Assessments	Priority Interventions	Outcome Criteria

Meds R/T to Concept:
Labs R/T to Concept:
Equipment R/T to Concept:
Client/Family Teaching R/T to Concept:

Bottom-right concept box

Concept:		
Outcome:		
System-Specific Assessments	Priority Interventions	Outcome Criteria

Meds R/T to Concept:
Labs R/T to Concept:
Equipment R/T to Concept:
Client/Family Teaching R/T to Concept:

To be completed and reviewed the day of clinical by: Clinical Instructor signature: _____ Date _____

Developed by Lydia R. Zager, MSN, RN, NEA-BC; Additions from Kate Chappell, MSN, APRN, CPNP

ADULT HEALTH CONCEPT MAP TOOL, PAGE 2

Name_____

Evaluation of Outcome Criteria:

Rationale for Interventions:

Client response to interventions:

Clinical Judgment. Was overall outcome met: Yes _____ Partially _____ Not at all _____
Rationale: Explain your decision. What would you do differently?

Evaluation of Outcome Criteria:

Rationale for Interventions:

Client response to interventions:

Clinical Judgment. Was overall outcome met: Yes _____ Partially _____ Not at all _____
Rationale: Explain your decision. What would you do differently?

Evaluation of Outcome Criteria:

Rationale for Interventions:

Client response to interventions:

Clinical Judgment. Was overall outcome met: Yes _____ Partially _____ Not at all _____
Rationale: Explain your decision. What would you do differently?

Priority Lab/Procedures	Results/Interpretations	Nursing Indications (Pre & Post)

AIDES MEDICATION INFORMATION TOOL

Directions: Please complete on _____ of your priority medications
Turn into clinical instructor _____
Have ready as information for all drugs you are administering (book, drug cards)

"AIDES" to Assist in Remembering Facts for Medication Administration

Name of Drug: Brand_____ **Generic**_____

Classification_____ **Referenced Used**_____

A	Action of medication:
	Administration of medication. Dosage ordered_____
	How to administer:
	Assessment:
	Adverse Effects. List significant ones:
	Accuracy/Appropriateness of order. Is it indicated based on client's condition, known allergies, drug-drug or drug-food interactions? If not, what action did you take?
I	Interactions (Drug-Drug, Food-Drug):
	Identify priority plan prior to giving drug (i.e., vital signs, labs, allergies, etc.):
	Identify priority plan after giving drug:
D	Desired outcomes of the drug:
	Discharge teaching—Administration considerations for client and family:
E	Evaluate signs and symptoms of complications. Intervene if necessary and describe:
S	Safety (client identification, risk for falls, vital sign assessments):

EXAMPLE OF REFLECTION QUESTIONS

Student Name _____ Clinical Instructor _____

Sec # _____ Date_____ Sat/UnSat or Grade_____

Date due to Clinical Instructor: _____

Six (6) points are possible and will be added to Rubric Grading Tool for the Concept Map (see Appendix B)

1. Connect the clinical findings (diagnostic test results) to the priority interventions (medications, treatments) for your client and provide the rationale. (2 points)

2. Based on your analysis of the concepts, what are the expected outcomes for your client?
   (2 points)

3. What went well today for you in clinical and why? (1 point)

4. What would you do differently and why? (1 point)

APPENDIX F

Chapter 4

HISTORY AND PATHOPHYSIOLOGY INFORMATION TOOL

Student Name _____ Faculty _____ Sec #_____

Date _____ Pass/Fail or Grade_____

Directions: Complete and submit to clinical instructor by _____.
(10 points possible on the Rubric Grading Tool for the Concept Map)

Client's Story (History)—What symptoms required the client to come to the hospital?

PATHOPHYSIOLOGY

Please describe the etiology (cause) and pathophysiology in your words. This is to be completed for the major diagnosis and any other active diagnoses that affect care (i.e., diabetes).

List the signs and symptoms of the disease from the textbook. Compare it to the clinical system specific assessment findings from your client (may complete the comparison after you care for your client during clinical).

Assessment findings (signs & symptoms) from textbook:	Assessment findings my client manifested:
_____	_____
_____	_____
_____	_____
_____	_____
_____	_____
_____	_____
_____	_____

HEALTH HISTORY AND SYSTEM-SPECIFIC ASSESSMENT TOOL	
Demographic Information	
Source of History	
Chief Concern/Complaint	
History of Present Illness (HPI)	
Past Medical History (PMH)	
Family History (FH)	
Social History (SH)	
Health Promotion Behaviors	
Review of Systems (ROS) System-Specific as indicated by client condition: • Integument • Head and Neck • Eyes • Ears, Nose, Mouth and Throat • Breasts • Respiratory • Cardiovascular • Gastrointestinal • Genitourinary • Musculoskeletal • Neurological • Mental Health • Endocrine • Allergic/Immunologic	
Focused History of Symptom(s) • Location • Quality • Quantity • Timing • Setting • Alleviating or Aggravating Factors • Associated Phenomenon	

Adapted by Ellen Synovec, MN

cont'd on next page

HEALTH HISTORY AND SYSTEM-SPECIFIC ASSESSMENT TOOL *(cont'd))*

II PHYSICAL ASSESSMENT

General Survey
1. Appearance
2. Level of Consciousness
3. Behavior/Affect
4. Posture/dress
5. Signs of discomfort or distress
6. Assess pupils for symmetry, shape, reactivity light

Skin Assessment:
1. Color
2. Condition—Look behind ears, skin folds, between toes, soles of feet, pressure areas on shoulder, sacrum, heels
   Presence or absence or lesions, scars, wounds or piercings
3. Texture
4. Temperature
5. Skin turgor sternum
6. Nails condition, presence of clubbing
7. Capillary refill bilaterally fingers

Respiratory Assessment
1. Rate
2. Rhythm
3. Accessory muscle use
4. Chest shape and symmetry/spinal deformities/AP: LA
5. Ausculation 12 sites anterior, posterior and axillary—assess for presence or absence of adventitious sounds, cough, congestion

Cardiac assessment
1. PMI—assess location and size
2. 4 auscultation sites with diaphragm and bell
   a. Aortic—2nd RICS RSB
   b. Pulmonic—2nd LICS LSB
   c. Tricuspid—4th LICS, along left lateral sternal border
   d. Mitral or apical pulse—5th LICS MCL, apex of heart
3. Carotids—assess pulse quality, presence or absence of thrills/bruits, bilaterally
4. JVD
5. Lymph nodes

Abdomen
1. Size
2. Shape
3. Symmetry
4. Condition—presence or absence of piercings, scars, striae, pulsations, peristalsis or bulges
5. Bowel sounds—assess all 4 quads, # sounds per minute RLQ
6. Assess for distention or tenderness with light palpation

Extremities
1. Capillary refill to upper extremities (UE)
2. Assess UE and lower extremities (LE) for general range of motion
3. Assess UE and LE for condition, color, temperature and presence of edema
4. Palpation of peripheral pulses—radial and dorsal pedalis
5. Assess clonus

Adapted by Ellen Synovec, MN

LAB AND DIAGNOSTIC TESTS AND PROCEDURES TOOL
Use as Reference for Client Care

Name: _____

Date: _____

Client Initials: _____

Directions: Identify only <u>pertinent</u> labs to the client condition, whether normal or abnormal. Describe what caused the client to have an abnormal lab or why a lab may now be normal (e.g., norm WBC−client on antibiotics). Also explain why you would or would not call the healthcare provider about this lab. These laboratory values may vary in textbooks. Look at the accepted norms for the institution where the test is interpreted to determine abnormal versus normal. This list is not all inclusive.

Lab Test	Date of Lab Test	Results	Normal	Pertinence to Client	Would You Call the Healthcare Provider?
Hematology					
WBC			5.0 − 10.0 10^3 ul		
RBC			4.2 − 5.4 10^6 µL		
HGB			12.0 − 16.0 g/dL		
HbA1c			6% or less		
HCT			37.0 − 47.0%		
MCV			81 − 89 µm³		
MCH			26 − 35 pg/cell		
MCHC			31 − 37 g/dl		
Platelets			150,000− 400,000/mm³		
Neutrophils			37 − 75%		
Lymphocytes			19 − 48%		
Monocytes			0 − 10%		
Eosinophils			1 − 3%		
Basophils			0.0 − 1.5%		
Chemistry					
Sodium			135 − 145 mEq/L		
Potassium			3.5 − 5.1 mEq/L		
Chloride			98 − 107 mEq/L		
Glucose−serum			70 − 110 mg/dL		
Magnesium			1.3 − 2.1 mEq/L		
BUN			6 − 20 mg/dL		
Creatinine			0.7 − 1.4 mg/dL		
Calcium			8.5 −11.0 mg/dL		
Protein			6.0 − 8.0 mg/dL		
Albumin			3.5 − 5.0 mg/dL		
A/G Ratio			1.5:1.0 − 2.5 :1.0		
Total Bilirubin			0.3 −1.3 mg/dL		
Direct bilirubin			0 − 0.4 mg/dL		
Indirect Bilirubin			0.2 − .8 mg/dL		
ALT, SGPT			10 − 30 U/L		
AST, SGOT			8 − 46 U/L		
Ammonia			80 − 110 dL/mcg		

cont'd on next page

APPENDIX H

LAB & DIAGNOSTIC TESTS AND PROCEDURES TOOL *(cont'd)*

Lab Test	Date of Lab Test	Results	Normal	Pertinence to Client	Would You Call the Healthcare Provider?
LDH – serum			91 – 180 mg/dL		
Alk Phos			35 – 142 U/L		
Uric Acid			2 – 7 mg/dL		
Phosphorus			2.5 – 4.5 mg/dL		
Total Cholesterol			< 200 mg/dL		
LDL age > 45 (LD)			90 – 185 mg/dL		
HDL			40 – 65 mg/dL		
Triglyceride			35 – 150 mg/dL		
Urinalysis					
Color			Clear Yellow		
Appearance			Clear		
Glucose			Neg.		
Bilirubin			Neg		
Ketones			Neg		
Specific Gravity			1.015 – 1.025		
Blood			Neg		
Ph			5 – 9		
Protein			Neg		
Urobilinogen			0.5 – 4.0 mg/24hr		
Nitrates			Neg		
ABG's					
pH			7.35 – 7.45		
pCO_2			35 – 45 mm Hg		
pO_2			80 – 100 mm Hg		
HCO_3			22 – 26 mEq /L		
O_2 Sat			> 95%		
Type of O_2 client receiving					
Digoxin			0.5 – 2.0 µg/mL		
Dilantin			10 – 20 µg/mL		
Tegretol			4 –12 µg/mL		
Theophylline			10 – 20 µg/mL		
Pt			12 – 14 SEC		
Ptt			30 – 45 SEC		
Amylase			25 – 125 U/dL		
Cardiac Enzymes					
Myoglobin			30 – 90 ng/mL		
Total CPK (CK)			Male 5 – 55 U/L Female 5 – 25 U/L		
CPK-MB			0 – 7% of total CPK		
CPK-BB			0% of total CPK		
CPK-MM			5 – 70% of total CPK		
Troponin I Value			< 0.6 ng/mL		
BNP			< 100 pg/mL		

LAB & DIAGNOSTIC TESTS AND PROCEDURES TOOL *(cont'd)*

DIAGNOSTIC TESTS/PROCEDURES

1. X-Ray, Endoscopy, Scans, Biopsy, C & S, or other special procedure reports

   Test: _____

   Date: _____

   Conclusion/Interpretations: _____

   _____

   _____

   Pertinence to Client: _____

2. X-Ray, Endoscopy, Scans, Biopsy, C&S, or other special procedure reports

   Test: _____

   Date: _____

   Conclusion/Interpretations: _____

   _____

   _____

   Pertinence to Client: _____

3. X-Ray, Endoscopy, Scans, Biopsy, C & S, or other special procedure reports

   Test: _____

   Date: _____

   Conclusion/Interpretations: _____

   _____

   _____

   Pertinence to Client: _____

APPENDIX I

Chapter 4

NURSING FOUNDATIONS/FUNDAMENTALS CONCEPT MAP TOOL

Name _____ Clinical Instructor _____ Sec # _____ Date _____

Grade _____

Concept:

Overall Outcome:

System-Specific Assessments	Priority Interventions	Outcome Criteria

Concept:

Overall Outcome:

System-Specific Assessments	Priority Interventions	Outcome Criteria

MEDICAL DIAGNOSIS & Pertinent History/Information

Client Age:

Height: Weight:

Allergies:

Meds R/T to Concept Above:

Labs/Diag. Tests for Above Concept:

Equipment/Risks/Precautions:

Meds R/T to Concept Above:

Labs/Diag. Tests for Above Concept:

Family Involvement Care/Client Teaching:

Adapted for Foundations by Kimberly Glenn, RN, MN, CPN

NURSING FOUNDATIONS/FUNDAMENTALS CONCEPT MAP TOOL, PAGE 2

Name

Evaluation of Outcome Criteria:

Rationale for Interventions:

Client response to interventions:

Clinical Judgment. Was overall outcome met: Yes _____   Partially _____   Not at all _____
Rationale: Explain your decision. What would you do differently?

Evaluation of Outcome Criteria:

Rationale for Interventions:

Client response to interventions:

Clinical Judgment. Was overall outcome met: Yes _____   Partially _____   Not at all _____
Rationale: Explain your decision. What would you do differently?

Adapted for Foundations by Kimberly Glenn, RN, MN, CPN

CHILDREN AND FAMILIES CONCEPT MAP TOOL

Name _____ Clinical Faculty _____ Clinical Date _____

Client Age:
Gender:
Height/length:
Weight:
Allergies:
Reason for admission:
Pertinent History/ Information:

Concept:
Overall Outcome:

System-Specific Assessments	Interventions	Outcome Criteria

Meds R/T Outcome Above:

Labs/Tests and Results for Above Outcome:

Lab values you would want, and why, if none obtained:

Concept:
Overall Outcome:

System-Specific Assessments	Interventions	Outcome Criteria

Meds R/T tOutcome Above:

Labs/Tests and Results for Above Outcome:

Lab values you would want, and why, if none obtained:

Concept:
Overall Outcome:

System-Specific Assessments	Interventions	Outcome Criteria

Meds R/T Outcome Above:

Labs/Tests and Results for Above Outcome:

Lab values you would want, and why, if none obtained:

Patient/Family Support and Teaching:

Equipment/Risks/Precautions:

Expected Piaget stage for age:
Your client's Piaget stage:
Expected Erikson stage for age:
Your client's Erikson stage:
Client's hourly fluid requirement (and calculation):

To be completed and verified the day of clinical by: Faculty signature:_____

Adapted by Kate K. Chappell, MSN, APRN, PHP-BC

CHILDREN AND FAMILIES CONCEPT MAP TOOL, PAGE 2

Name_____

Concept:

Evaluation of Outcome Criteria:

Rationale for Interventions:

Client response to interventions:

Clinical Judgment. Was overall outcome met: Yes_____ Partially_____ Not at all_____

Rationale: Explain your decision. What would you do differently?

Concept:

Evaluation of Outcome Criteria:

Rationale for Interventions:

Client response to interventions:

Clinical Judgment. Was overall outcome met: Yes_____ Partially_____ Not at all_____

Rationale: Explain your decision. What would you do differently?

Adapted for Pediatrics by Kate Chappell, MSN, APRN, PNP- BC

APPENDIX K

Chapter 4

MATERNAL AND NEWBORN CONCEPT MAP TOOL

Name _____ Clinical Instructor _____ Clinical Unit _____ Date of Care _____

Concept:
Overall Outcome:

Medical Dx & Pertinent History/ Information:

Client's age:
Allergies:
Ht:
Wt:

Meds R/T Outcomes:

Labs/Procedures R/T Outcomes:

Pt / Family Support & Teaching:

Risks/Precautions/Equipment:

Concept:
Overall Outcome:

System-Specific Assessments Data/Risk Factors	Interventions	Outcome Criteria

Concept:
Overall Outcome:

System-Specific Assessments Data/Risk Factors	Interventions	Outcome Criteria

Adapted for OB by Eileen Leaphart RN, MN and Heather Schneider, MSN, RN-BC

MATERNAL AND NEWBORN CONCEPT MAP TOOL, PAGE 2

Nursing Concept #1
Evaluation of Outcome Criteria:

Rationale for Interventions:

Client response to interventions:

Clinical Judgment Was overall outcome met: Yes _____   Partially _____   Not at all _____
Rationale: Explain your decision. What would you do differently?

Nursing Concept #2
Evaluation of Outcome Criteria:

Rationale for Interventions:

Client response to interventions:

Clinical Judgment. Was overall outcome met: Yes _____   Partially _____   Not at all _____
Rationale: Explain your decision. What would you do differently?

Adapted for OB by Eileen Leaphart RN, MN and Heather Schneider, MSN, RN-BC

APPENDIX L

Chapter 4

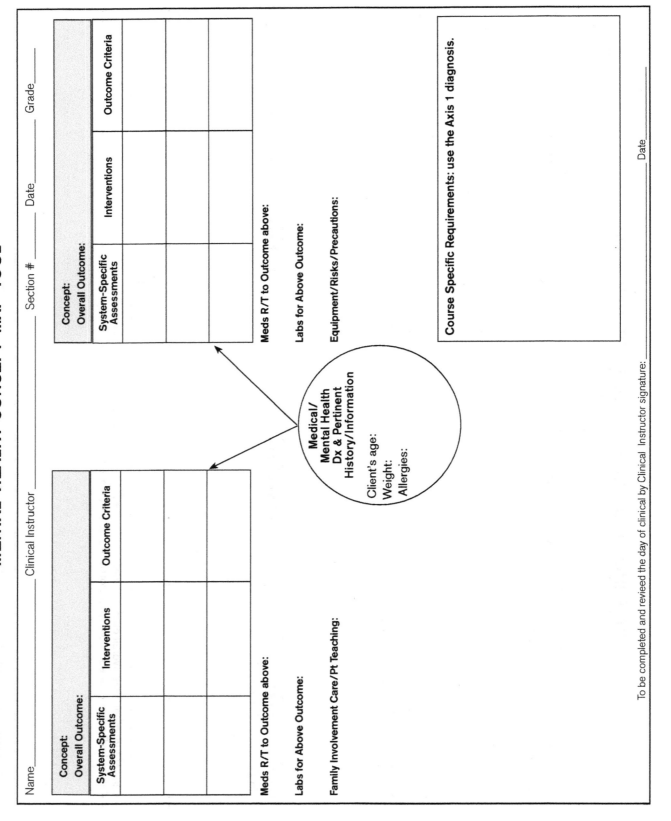

MENTAL HEALTH CONCEPT MAP TOOL

Name_____ Clinical Instructor_____ Section #_____ Date_____ Grade_____

Concept:
Overall Outcome:

System-Specific Assessments	Interventions	Outcome Criteria

Meds R/T to Outcome above:

Labs for Above Outcome:

Family Involvement Care/Pt Teaching:

Concept:
Overall Outcome:

System-Specific Assessments	Interventions	Outcome Criteria

Meds R/T to Outcome above:

Labs for Above Outcome:

Equipment/Risks/Precautions:

Medical/
Mental Health
Dx & Pertinent
History/Information

Client's age:
Weight:
Allergies:

Course Specific Requirements: use the Axis 1 diagnosis.

To be completed and revieed the day of clinical by Clinical Instructor signature:_____ Date_____

MENTAL HEALTH CONCEPT MAP TOOL, PAGE 2

Evaluation of Outcome Criteria:	Rationale for Interventions:	Client response to interventions:

Clinical Judgment. Was overall outcome met: Yes _____   Partially _____   Not at all _____
Rationale: Explain your decision. What would you do differently?

Evaluation of Outcome Criteria:	Rationale for Interventions:	Client response to interventions:

Clinical Judgment. Was overall outcome met: Yes _____   Partially _____   Not at all _____
Rationale: Explain your decision. What would you do differently?

Evaluation of Outcome Criteria:	Rationale for Interventions:	Client response to interventions:

Clinical Judgment. Was overall outcome met: Yes _____   Partially _____   Not at all _____
Rationale: Explain your decision. What would you do differently?

Priority Lab/Procedures	Results/Interpretations	Nursing Indications (Pre & Post)

ENGAGING THE LEARNER ACTIVITIES

STUDENT-CENTERED LEARNING ACTIVITIES
LINKED TO PROFESSIONAL AND NCLEX® STANDARDS

Resources Needed for Activities	*Nursing Made Insanely Easy!* (Manning & Zager, 2014); *The Eight-Step Approach for Teaching Clinical Nursing* (Zager, Manning & Herman, 2017)	*Concepts Made Insanely Easy for Clinical Nursing* (Manning & Zager, 2014); *The Eight-Step Approach for Student Clinical Success* (Zager, Manning & Herman, 2017)
Standards	**Faculty Instructions**	**Student Instructions**

Management of Care
 	
Plan, implement, and evaluate client-centered care based on Standards of Practice.
	Steps in Constructing the Concept Map
	(Refer to Chapter 4)
	
	Recommended for 1st clinical course, lab or simulation. Activities can be adapted based on the level of the student.
	
	1. Explain the steps as the students construct a concept map using the example given in the book.
	
	   a. Have the students go step by step as listed in the book.
	
	   b. Answer questions the students have about constructing the concept map.
		Steps in Constructing the Concept Map
		(Refer to Chapter 4 and *Concepts Made Insanely Easy for Clinical Nursing* for concepts, assessments, and expected outcomes)
		
		1. Construct a concept map.
		
		   a. Proceed step by step as listed in the book.
		
		   b. Ask questions as needed about the steps as you construct the concept map.

Management of Care
 	
Plan, implement, and evaluate client-centered care based on Standards of Practice.
	Concept Map Practice
	(Refer students to the blank Concept Map Tool, end of chapter 4, The *Eight-Step Approach for Student Clinical Success* and the book *Concepts Made Insanely Easy for Clinical Nursing* for concepts, assessments, and expected outcomes)
	
	2. Have the students with a partner, construct a concept map based on another disease or pathophysiological process. Have students:
	
	   a. Hypothesize possible concepts related to the pathophysiology of the disease process.
	
	   b. Determine what assessments would confirm or reject their hypothesized concepts.
	
	   c. Select the priority interventions after they analyze the concepts.
	
	   d. Determine the outcome criteria that would indicate their client has met the expected outcomes.
		Concept Map Practice
		(Refer to end of Chapter 4 for Blank Concept Map Tool and the book *Concepts Made Insanely Easy for Clinical Nursing* for concepts, assessments, and expected outcomes)
		
		2. Based on the assigned disease or pathophysiological process, construct a concept map with your partner.
		
		   a. Hypothesize possible concepts related to the pathophysiology of the disease process.
		
		   b. Determine what assessments would confirm or reject your hypothesized concepts.
		
		   c. Select the priority interventions after you analyze the concepts.
		
		   d. Determine the outcome criteria that would indicate your client has met the expected outcomes.

Components of Successful Simulation

Erin McKinney, MN, RN, RNC-OB / Kate K. Chappell, MSN, APRN, CPNP-PC

IN THIS CHAPTER YOU WILL LEARN ABOUT:

➞ Preplanning for simulation

➞ Planning for simulation

➞ Designing the scenario

➞ Staging the simulation/scenario

➞ Preparing the simulation team

➞ Running the scenario

➞ Debriefing the scenario

➞ Evaluating the team and the simulation experience

INTRODUCTION

Simulation is a part of every nursing education program in some format. "Simulation education is a bridge between classroom learning and real-life clinical experience" (Simulation for Society in Healthcare, 2016). The purpose of simulation is to provide an opportunity for authentic learning where the student can perform aspects of client care without risk to the client, receive feedback, and be able to perform the care again. Purposeful simulation should be standards-based and curriculum-driven! An excellent resource to solidify their skills is the International Nursing Association for Clinical Simulation and Learning (INACSL) which developed the INACSL Standards of Best Practice: Simulation^SM. The standards are posted on the INACSL website and can be downloaded for free. The INACSL Standards of Best Practice were designed to advance the science of simulation, share best practices, and provide evidence based guidelines for implementation and training. However, conducting an effective and efficient simulation experience for students can be very challenging.

Simulation is an ideal platform for illustrating the standards of practice and the priorities of safe and effective patient care. The standards and the priorities must guide the simulation team in their selection of scenarios from the curriculum that prepares the student while they are in school. Simulation also prepares students for clinical practice after graduation. Simulation requires preplanning with all of the team members involved.

PREPLANNING FOR SIMULATION

There are important decisions and factors that the college/school of nursing and curriculum committee need to consider prior to planning simulation.

1. Determine if your state board of nursing has a policy on how many simulation hours can replace clinical hours.

2. The curriculum committee members must decide how much simulation may be used to replace clinical hours in your curriculum within the guidelines of your state board of nursing.

   ✦ The clinical simulation ratio supported in the literature is 1:1 or 2:1 ratio (Hayden, Smiley, Alexander, Kardong-Edgren, & Jeffries, 2014). Either is a satisfactory ratio when the experience is well planned and implemented and the downtime for students is minimal.

   ✦ A four-hour slot would be equal to an eight-hour clinical day if you chose 2:1 ratio. During that time, you could provide a preconference, 2 scenarios and a skill station. If you have two simulation rooms, you could accommodate 24 students.

3. Determine the type(s) of manikins you have for simulation experiences (Refer to Appendix A–**Example of Adapting a Scenario to High, Moderate and Low Fidelity Manikins**):

   ✦ **High Fidelity**— "Experiences using full scale computerized patient simulators, virtual reality or standardized patients that are extremely realistic and provide a high level of interactivity and realism for the learner" (NLN-SIRC, 2013, p. S-6).

   ✦ **Moderate or Mid-Fidelity**—"Experiences that are more technologically sophisticated such as computer-based self-directed learning systems simulations in which the participant relies on a two-dimensional focused experience to problem solve, perform a skill, and make decisions or the use of manikins more realistic than static low fidelity ones having breath sounds, heart sounds and/or pulses" (NLN-SIRC, 2013, p. S-7).

   ✦ **Low Fidelity**—"Experiences such as case studies, role-playing, using partial task trainers or static manikins to immerse students in a clinical situation or practice a specific skill" (NLN-SIRC, 2013, p. S-7).

   ✦ **Task Trainers**—"Simulators that are used to practice a skill such as an IV arm that is used to practice IV insertions skills" (Kardong-Edgren, et al., 2011, p. S4–S5).

4. Determine if you have the scenarios you need for simulation.

   ✦ There are numerous sources for free scenarios or for purchase (Refer to Appendix B—**Where to Find Free Simulations**).

   ✦ There are templates available to guide original scenario development including National League for Nursing (NLN) as well as others (Refer to Appendix C—**Scenario Design Template**).

✦ Original scenarios may be needed when you cannot find what you need. For example, if you need a scenario to ensure students are ready to respond to pediatric or adult emergencies prior to clinical, please refer to Appendix D–**Example of an Original Scenario Packet: Pediatric Emergency Response** and Appendix E– **Example of an Original Scenario Packet: Adult Respiratory Distress Due to Hypovolemia.**

The *Original Scenario Example Packet* contains all of the documents needed to run the scenario. This is very helpful as often the facilitators have not reviewed the materials prior to the day of the simulation. *The packet will save the day! We recommend labeling the packet as "Desk Copy–DO NOT REMOVE" to prevent it being removed from the lab.*

5. Determine how orientation will be done for faculty members participating in simulation. The orientation should be held at the beginning of the semester to include:

   ✦ Participating in the scenario in a student role.

   ✦ Running the scenario as a facilitator to become comfortable with the software, and conducting an educationally sound debrief.

   ✦ Prior to the orientation, faculty should review the information. One effective method is to provide an orientation course and materials through an online course management system (i.e., Blackboard). (Refer to Appendix F— **Screenshot of Online Orientation Course**).

6. Determine how orientation will be done for students participating in simulation. Plan orientation in every course throughout their nursing education. A course management system (i.e., Blackboard) can be used for orientation. It can be used to:

   ✦ Introduce the students to the lab, the manikins, medication dispensing machine, and available equipment.

   ✦ Post student weekly objectives and assignments for the coming simulation.

   ✦ Post other valuable resources for the students (Refer to Appendix G—**Helpful Tips When Doing Simulation**).

The rest of this chapter is organized with tables, each reflecting key components for a successful simulation.

   ✦ Table 1: Planning the Simulation

   ✦ Table 2: Designing the Scenario

   ✦ Table 3: Staging the Simulation/Scenario

   ✦ Table 4: Preparing the Simulation Team

   ✦ Table 5: Running the Scenario

   ✦ Table 6: Debriefing the Scenario

   ✦ Table 7: Evaluating the Team and Simulation Experience

Now that the preplanning decisions are made, you are ready to plan the simulation. Table 1 will guide you in planning your simulation.

TABLE 1: PLANNING THE SIMULATION

Planning the Simulation	Strategies	Comments/Suggestions
• Planning Meeting (i.e., course coordinators, clinical faculty and simulation director, etc.)	Meeting Materials: • Semester calendar for the course • Semester calendar for the simulation lab • List of available scenarios already developed (or template for scenario creation)	• The planning meeting with all involved team members is essential for successful simulation. • The course calendar guides team members to focus on the concepts based on standards in the course curriculum that should be emphasized in the simulation scenario. • Simulations should follow the curriculum lecture schedule so the student will have content exposure prior to simulation.
• Simulation Scheduling (Refer to Appendix H–Template for Scheduling Simulation and Skill Stations)	• Place the necessary blocks of time for the group simulation on the simulation lab schedule and in the course syllabus. • Do this for each simulation day needed. • Calculate the time needed for each team to run the simulation, debrief the simulation and setup the room prior to the next group run. • When a skill station runs concurrently with a simulation, the skill station activities must be tailored to fit the time allotted for the simulation.	• The day is typically divided into one-hour blocks. • The simulation (15 mins) and debrief (45 mins) takes an hour per group of eight. (Refer to Appendix I–Example of Clinical Day Simulation and Skill Station Schedule) • Debrief lasts approximately 2 to 3 times as long as the scenario. (See Table 6 Debriefing the Scenario in this chapter) • On average 15 minutes is plenty of simulation time if your goals and objectives are focused. • If your group is small, run two students at a time rather than four. • If time is limited, debrief does not have to follow every group's simulation. Debrief can be done after every 2nd or 4th group. While other simulation teams are participating in the simulation, the waiting students can practice at skill stations or review case studies that are not tied to the scenario. They may also complete their concept map based on the scenario. This makes the waiting time productive versus social media time!

When the coordination described in Table 1 is completed, you are ready to design the scenario. Table 2 will take you through the steps of creating a scenario that is matched to the standards in your curriculum.

TABLE 2: DESIGNING THE SCENARIO

Designing the Scenario	Strategies	Comments/Suggestions

Scenario Design	• The scenario is designed based on where the student is in the curriculum (i.e., first, middle or last course, etc.).
	• Keep the goals of the scenario to one or two specific tasks and/or concepts.
	• Using a standard scenario (Refer to Appendix C– Scenario Design Template) helps in designing scenarios with consistency.
		• A scenario with too many "problems" will be difficult to complete in the allotted time.
		• Example of a scenario focus could be fluid and electrolytes. The scenario would have:
		  • Focused assessment by the student (i.e. vital signs and pertinent lab results).
		  • The need to call a healthcare provider with an SBAR report.
		  • A specific set of received orders to bolus the client, adjust IV flow rate following the bolus and reassess vital signs.

Scenario Selection (Refer to Appendix B–Where to Find Free Simulations; and the Reference List at the end of the book)	• A scenario designed for fluid and electrolyte concepts must clearly focus on fluid overload or fluid deficit. • Be sure that all aspects of the scenario match the goals of the simulation.	• A practice exercise with the faculty that are running the simulation is highly recommended. • The practice ensures that all aspects of the experience are accurate, evidence-based, meet course goals and can be completed in the designated time planned.
• Skill Station or Activity Selection (i.e., running concurrently with the simulation). (Refer to Appendix I–Example of Clinical Day Simulation and Skill Station Schedule)	• The focus of the skill station needs to be related to the concepts in the scenario chosen. • If the information in the skill station is needed for the simulation, then it needs to be covered with assigned material prior to the simulation.	• The schedule for the day is more efficient when some clinical groups are at a skill station while others are doing simulation. • You may require pre simulation assignments, materials or other resources that help students prepare for the content of the scenario. **Example: Fluid and Electrolytes Skill Stations** • Station on urinalysis values. • Station with cups of yellow dyed water reflecting the range of urine concentrations. • Station for assessment of signs and symptoms of fluid volume deficit and excess.

Designing the simulation, as outlined in Table 2, describes the essential steps necessary to achieve the desired educational outcomes. The next component is setting the stage.

TABLE 3: STAGING THE SIMULATION/SCENARIO

Staging the Simulation/ Scenario	Strategies	Comments/Suggestions
Simulation Lab Setup (Refer to Appendix J– Template for Simulation Lab Setup)	• Stage the client room as realistically as possible (i.e., actual hand washing, availability of gloves, applying oxygen, administering injections into IV tubing or an injection pad taped to a manikin, etc.). • Provide clipboard with provider orders and medication administration record unless you have an Electronic Medical Record (EMR).	• Realism in simulation helps bridge the gap between the simulation world and the real clinical world. • Use wigs, glasses, hats, clothes, pictures of wounds laminated and applied to client, bruises using pink and blue eye shadow, etc. • Use props as appropriate: incentive spirometer, tissues, emesis basin, urinal, etc. **Helpful Hints:** • The best time to collect items for simulation is right after Halloween! • For olfactory staging, use ammonia for elevated ammonia levels, old cigarettes for smoking, something with strong sweet odor for ketoacidosis, V8 or egg white with food coloring for gastrointestinal drainage. There are books on how to do moulage, kits available for purchase, or use your creative imagination!
Programming the Scenario	• If you have a high-fidelity manikin it is ideal to program a change in physiologic states that are linked to the expected intervention by the student. • For example, an increase in the blood pressure and a decrease in heart rate after providing a fluid bolus for symptoms of fluid volume deficit. • If you have a moderate (mid) fidelity manikin you may change the state using the remote or the SimPad. • If you are using low fidelity, then laminated vital sign cards may be handed to the students at the appropriate time. (Refer to Appendix A, Example of Adapting a Scenario to High, Moderate and Low Fidelity Manikins)	• When you design a scenario, anticipate that some teams will provide proper interventions that were intended, but you may get a wide range of responses from the students that were not intended. • Let the scenario continue, even if the intended response/interventions by the student does not occur. Resist the temptation to lead the students toward the intended goal. Critical points related to the goal should be discussed during the debrief. (Refer to Table 6–Debriefing the Scenario for examples of correct and incorrect actions taken by the students) • Students may not perform the proper interventions during the simulation. When this occurs, the client labs, vital signs, etc. should reflect a decline in client status or lack of improvement. • The participants are encouraged to think independently. • Facilitators should avoid prompting and directives during the scenario.

TABLE 3: STAGING THE SIMULATION/SCENARIO *(cont'd)*

Staging the Simulation/ Scenario	Strategies	Comments/Suggestions
Staffing for the day	• The simulation facilitator should be the person who performs the debrief. • You can always run two simulation rooms, then, debrief all the students together at the end if time is limited. • Additional 1-2 faculty members will be needed to run each skill station or you can design a station with clear objectives that students can run independently. • Examples of skill stations are provided in Chapter 6. (Refer to Chapter 6, Appendix E–Pediatric Growth Assessment and Appendix F–Medication Administration Skill Station)	• The course faculty leader needs to clearly define the scenario objectives and roles for each faculty member involved in the simulation. • An organized simulation day makes for a smooth teaching and learning experience. (Students and faculty that are assisting benefit from a structured organized experience.) • Post instructions and prep information for the simulation on your communication board at least 2 days prior to the simulation day. • Project the daily schedule onto a screen or whiteboard for visibility throughout the day. (Refer to Appendix I, Example of Clinical Day Simulation Schedule)

Table 3 described how you can create authenticity in your stimulation. Table 4 outlines how to prepare the simulation team.

TABLE 4: PREPARING THE SIMULATION TEAM

Preparing the Simulation Team	Strategies	Comments/Suggestions

Facilitator Guide
 	
(Refer to Appendix K—Example of Faculty Simulation Guide)
	• The faculty leader should notify adjunct faculty of the schedule and the materials needed for the simulation.
	
	• This preparation is essential for an organized simulation.
	
	• During the simulation, the facilitator may use a faculty guide (Refer to Appendix K—Example of Faculty Simulation Guide) or a grading rubric to evaluate the performance of the student. Use one form for each simulation.
	
	• The notes recorded by the facilitator on the guide will be helpful when discussing teaching points during the debrief.
	
	• Provide materials to guide the facilitator and standardize the experience from one team to the next (Refer to Appendix D—Example of an Original Scenario Packet: Pediatric Emergency Response). The packet contains:
	  • Client report
	  • Scenario script for facilitator
	  • Provider orders
	  • Medication Administration Record
	  • Healthcare provider orders (i.e. telephone orders if the student calls the provider)
	  • Debrief guidelines
	  • Grading rubric (if graded) or the Faculty guide (if not graded)
	
	Skill Station Materials:
	Provide laminated faculty bullet points to assist with running the skill station. This helps with consistency of the skill station from one faculty member to another.
		• Make sure all facilitators understand the objectives of the simulation and skill stations before the start of the simulation day.
		
		• The script for the scenario should include all anticipated responses for the client (i.e., "My pain is bad," moaning, noisy respirations, etc.).
		
		• Responses for assessment information not obtainable from assessing the manikin must be scripted (i.e., skin temp and color, pitting edema, status of IV site, etc.).
		
		• Faculty must use the approved script to ensure the simulation is consistent from one time to the next and each student receives the same information.

A well prepared simulation team helps ensure an organized, consistent, and educationally sound simulation. Now that the preparation is done, Table 5 will guide the process of implementation.

TABLE 5: RUNNING THE SCENARIO

Running the Scenario	Strategies	Comments/Suggestions
Scenario Orchestration	• Create and distribute the simulation schedule that outlines the rotations of the students through the simulation(s) and/or skill stations. • Provide the client report to the student simulation team or provide the report to the entire group at the beginning of the day. • Run the simulation scenario. The assigned group of students participates in the simulation while the remaining students observe when the scenario is not graded. The participants and the observers debrief as a group. The facilitator who ran the scenario should debrief. (Refer to Appendix M–Worksheet for Debriefing for Meaningful Learning (DML) • Assign a designated person to re-set the stage to the start position between scenarios for the next group of students (i.e., removing the oxygen, pulse oximeter, straightening covers, changing the flow rate on IV, etc.).	• Scheduling requires coordination. (Refer to Appendix I–Example of Clinical Day Simulation and Skill Station Schedule) • Giving report to the entire group saves time but would not be appropriate if the simulation is graded. • The scenarios typically last 15–20 minutes with four student roles (i.e., 2 RNS, 1–2 family roles and an occasional observer). • If time allows, repeating the scenario with the same student team reinforces learning. • The students not participating in the simulation observe the scenario in a separate or observation room via live video. This helps keep the observers engaged and on task. The observers can use their recorded observations from the sheet when they participate in the debrief. (Refer to Appendix L–Simulation Observer's Worksheet) • When the team moves to their next scenario, the four students who observed the prior experience would take on simulation roles for the new scenario. • When you are planning, don't forget that re-setting the stage and getting students to and from the scenarios takes time.

A schedule is essential for an organized simulation experience as illustrated in Table 5. Trust us, without a schedule, chaos will occur and the educational experience will be less effective. Table 6 will describe one of the most important components of simulation, the debrief.

TABLE 6: DEBRIEFING THE SCENARIO

Debriefing the Scenario	Strategies	Comments/Suggestions
Debriefing	• Move students to a comfortable room with a white board. • Remind the students that debrief is confidential and should not be shared outside of the session. (Refer to Appendix N– Consent for Simulation Lab) • Laminate the 3 debrief (DML) questions and tape them to the top of the whiteboards. (Refer to Appendix M– Worksheet for Debriefing for Meaningful Learning [DML]) • Give students 3 to 4 minutes to answer the 3 questions on a sheet of paper. • All students participate by sharing their answers and comments to each question. • As a teaching moment, clarify any points of confusion and gaps in knowledge if they were noted but not addressed during the "three question" discussion.	Debrief Questions: 1. What is the first thing that comes to mind about the simulation experience? 2. What went well and why? 3. What would you do differently and why? (Dreifuerst, 2009 & 2012) • Positive reinforcement and feedback helps to encourage group discussion of each question. • Debriefing is a time of learning and reflection. It must remain positive and not negative or punitive. It should last approximately three times as long as the scenario. ***Examples of Feedback:*** **Positive feedback:** talking about what the students did well, the decisions, the actions, communication and teamwork. **Negative feedback:** shaming, singling out a student, embarrassing them on what they did wrong or mentioning inappropriate behavior observed during the simulation. • If there was a critical error made during the simulation (i.e., omission, medication error, etc.) have a private conversation with the team. It is important not to single out a specific individual or team during a group debrief.

TABLE 6: DEBRIEFING THE SCENARIO *(cont'd)*

Debriefing the Scenario	Strategies	Comments/Suggestions
	• The conclusion of the debrief includes discussion of the reflection points (DML) for the specific scenario: • **Thinking-in-action** (thinking that occurs during the simulation) • **Thinking-on-action** (thinking that occurs while reflecting after the simulation) • **Thinking-beyond-action** (thinking of how the experience will apply to future client's clinical situations) (Dreifuerst, 2009 & 2012)	• **Example:** Goal of the scenario was to recognize and respond to an Allergic Reaction. • **The Correct Action** was to recognize the client had a Cephlasporin allergy and that Rocephin was hanging. The student was to: a. Turn off the Rocephin. b. Provide O_2. c. Obtain emergency orders from the healthcare provider. • **The Incorrect Path** taken by the student during the simulation: a. The students confused stridor for wheezing and decided that the client was having an asthma attack. b. The students left the Rocephin hanging. c. The students provided O_2. d. The students called the healthcare provider for bronchodilators and aerosol treatments commonly used with asthma. An example of the three questions where the goal of the scenario was to recognize and respond to an allergic reaction: • **Thinking-in-action:** What system specific assessments based on the pathophysiology distinguish stridor from wheezing? • **Thinking-on-action:** Given a client has stridor, what are the priority interventions? • **Thinking-beyond-action:** For future clients with respiratory problems, it will be important to consider all potential options that are contributing to the client's status.

Debrief is absolutely essential for student learning to take place. Debriefing reinforces appropriate clinical decisions and illustrates the gaps in knowledge. Just as feedback is essential for the students, the evaluation of the simulation and the team members helps ensure the desired outcomes of the simulation are met. Table 7 will guide you through the evaluation process.

TABLE 7: EVALUATING THE TEAM AND THE SIMULATION EXPERIENCE

Evaluating the Team and the Simulation Experience	Strategies	Comments/Suggestions
Evaluation (Refer to Appendix O–Simulation Experience Survey for Students and Appendix P–Faculty Simulation Orientation Survey).	Provide time for participants and facilitators to evaluate the experience in a timely manner.	• Feedback should drive possible changes in your design of the scenario for the next time. • There will always be room for changes and improvements based on student and faculty observations. • A survey for evaluation with handheld electronic devices (i.e., iPad or surface pro, etc.) at the end of the session is an efficient way to get students/faculty responses and feedback. • It is important to evaluate the student and faculty performances to maintain the standards of your simulation program.

CONCLUSION

Simulation, as illustrated in the seven tables, requires extensive preparation, coordination, and clearly-stated, expected student outcomes for a positive learning experience. Unplanned simulation will not give you the outcomes you want! In order for maximal student learning to occur, the simulation has to be well organized with measurable student learning outcomes developed by the faculty before the simulation. The optimal benefit of simulation is to reinforce clinical decision-making in a safe environment. It provides a level of feedback that is difficult to achieve during a normal day in a clinical setting.

EXAMPLE OF ADAPTING A SCENARIO TO
HIGH, MODERATE, AND LOW-FIDELITY MANIKINS

REPORT FOR STUDENTS ON CLIENT LONNIE JOSEPH

Lonnie Joseph is a 46-year-old male who was admitted to our unit via the ED. He presented with a cough, congestion, chest pressure, and elevated temperature. Chest X-ray revealed RLL pneumonia. An IV was started with LR and is running at 100 mL/hour. He is receiving oxygen via simple mask. It has improved his O_2 saturation from 89% to 93%. He was given 600 mg of Ibupropen in the ED for a temperature of 102.1°F. His first dose of Cefoxitin came up from the pharmacy and it has been hung.

Manikin Adaptations	Low Fidelity	Moderate Fidelity	High Fidelity
Suction and Oxygen with simple mask	Nonfunctioning Headwall	Nonfunctioning Headwall	Functioning Headwall
Hospital Room Props	Bed, bedside table, over bed table	Bed, bedside table, over bed table	Bed, bedside table, over bed table
Bedside Record	Clipboard with Paper MAR and Orders	Clipboard with Paper MAR and Orders	Clipboard with Paper MAR and Orders or Electronic Medical Record
Client Manikin	Static Manikin or Standard Patient (SP)(Human)	Moderate fidelity manikin in hospital gown or SP	High fidelity manikin in hospital gown or SP
IV Pump with IV mini bag of Antibiotic	Pump with two bags (1000 mL and 50mL Rocephin)	Pump with two bags (1000 mL and 50 mL Rocephin)	Pump with two bags (1000 mL and 50 mL Rocephin)
Client Status Changes	Provide sets of vital signs on laminated cards with options for improvement and deterioration depending on student intervention actions. Use YouTube or recording of progressing anaphylactic breath sounds as client deteriorates. Have normal breath sounds recorded for client that improves with implemented interventions.	Set manikin VS and breath sounds as normal for beginning state. Make VS and breath sound adjustments for manikin according to student actions to reflect deterioration and/or improvement.	Programmed: all vital sign changes, breathing transitions from normal breath sounds to wheezes to stridor, other symptoms related to anaphylaxis programmed over 10 to 15 minutes. Intervention actions should be linked to changes in manikin state.
Facilitator Roles Stay in one of the roles (i.e., client or healthcare provider). Avoid directing the scenario.	Client and Healthcare Provider (follow set script).	Client and Healthcare Provider (follow set script).	Client and Healthcare Provider (follow set script).
Facilitator Position	Stay behind two-way mirror or screen.	Stay behind two-way mirror or screen.	In control room, stay behind two-way mirror or screen, monitor view of simulation room.
Voice of Client	Facilitator	Facilitator	Facilitator
Debrief by Facilitator	Debrief room or classroom	Debrief room or classroom	Debrief room or classroom

APPENDIX B

WHERE TO FIND FREE SIMULATION SCENARIOS

American Association of Medical Colleges. (2013). MedEd PORTAL.
https://www.mededportal.org/

Several resources, search for simulation scenarios. Designed for residents and med students. Scenarios reflect the lifespan (newborn to elderly), including decompensating pediatric patient (4 unfolding scenarios from osteomyelitis to septic shock), pneumothorax, pneumonia, cardiac tamponade, dental office emergencies, "a night on call", interprofessional communication skills, neutropenic fever/sepsis, and palliative care encounters. Most scenarios are peer reviewed.

California State University. (2013). Multimedia Educational Resource for Learning and Online Teaching (MERLOT).
http://www.merlot.org/merlot/index.htm

Learning materials from several disciplines. Simulations range from low fidelity to high fidelity scenarios as well as learning materials that can be used as adjunct in the classroom.

Center for Health Science interprofessional Education, Research and Practice. (2017). Scenario Building & Library.
http://collaborate.uw.edu/educators-toolkit/scenario-building-library.html-0

Template for scenario development and examples of building a scenario. Ideas for building a simulation curriculum and a scenario storyboarding tool. Scenario library includes acute pharyngitis, post-op bladder distention, wound care, respiratory distress. The full website contains other information on interprofessional team training, debriefing tools, error disclosure training, etc.

Health Simulation. (2012). Healthy Simulation Free Resources.
http://healthysimulation.com/316/greatplaces-to-get-free-simulation-scenarios/

Several resources, free scenarios, links to conferences (some free), product reviews. Newsletter available for free. Specifically had one page on designing pre-hospital medical simulation scenarios.

Kansas Board of Nursing. (2009). Simulation scenario library.
http://www.ksbn.org/cne/SimulationScenarioLibrary.htm

Developed by faculty at schools of nursing for nursing and other health programs. Scenarios include: GI bleed, femur fracture, head injury, heart failure, pediatric (nursing and/or respiratory therapy), basic, intermediate and complex medical/surgical. Pre-scenario worksheet is also provided. Consistent template with objectives, history and information, orders, supplies needed, medications, simulator set up, events, competencies, prompting question, and debriefing topics.

Minnesota Simulation Health Education Partnership (MSHEP). (2017). Minnesota Healthcare Simulation Library.
http://www.healthforceminnesota.org/simulation/

Requires registration (free). Simulation scenario library and blogs/discussions. Update in progress. Potential for new website URL in near future. Group is planning to use webinars to meet and discuss current trends in simulation education across Minnesota.

WHERE TO FIND FREE SIMULATION SCENARIOS *(cont'd)*

National League for Nursing. (2011). Faculty Resources: ACES: Advancing care excellence for seniors.
http://www.nln.org/facultyprograms/facultyresources/aces/index.htm

ACES contains, among other tools, unfolding cases related to care of seniors. They combine storytelling and simulation. There are audio clips, scenarios and tips for implementation.

National League for Nursing. (2013). Simulation Innovation Resource Center (SIRC).
http://sirc.nln.org/

Courses for designing, developing simulations, debriefing guidelines. Integration and evaluation suggestions. Discussion blogs related to research, equipment issues, faculty development, and inter-professional education. Requires login (free). Several scenarios for purchase in the SimStore (Laerdal).

Reid, C. & Raleigh, R. (2013). Where to find simulations free.
https://www.scribd.com/document/299632811/Where-to-Find-Simulation-Scenarios

Society for Academic Emergency Medicine. (2007). Simulation case library.
http://www.emedu.org/simlibrary/default.aspx?AspxAutoDetectCookieSupport=1

Developed by emergency physicians, peer reviewed scenarios include intentional overdose, epidural hematoma with coma, APAP overdose, massive hemoptysis, demonic possession. Medical based, but detailed information on signs, symptoms and medical management.

The Sim Tech. (2017). Scenarios.
http://thesimtech.com/scenarios/

Text document outlining a variety of simulation topics, learning objectives (KSA), scenario summary, environment details, instructions for personnel (confederates and not), manikin settings, scenario progression/script, and debriefing notes in downloadable format. Topics include dyspnea (asthma and pulmonary edema), hypertension (aortic dissection and autonomic dysreflexia), and burn (meth lab explosion.

(Reid & Raleigh, 2013)

APPENDIX C

Chapter 5

SCENARIO DESIGN TEMPLATE

Simulation Scenario Course Name	
Concepts: Client Name:	Learning Objectives: 1. 2. 3.

Placement in the Curriculum	
Low Stakes	High Stakes
Psychomotor Skills:	Cognitive Skills:

Brief Overview and Goals of Simulation for Faculty Preparation		
Pre-Briefing Time: (Example 15 min)	Simulation Time: (Example 30 min)	Debriefing Time: (Example 40-60 min)
Student Pre-Simulation Work:	Student Configuration	Orientation to the Unit
Primary Medical Diagnosis with Associated Co-Morbidities; Current Surgeries and/or Procedures	Report to Students	Report from Outgoing Nurse

Simulation—Client Care				
Time	Manikin Settings & Changes	Student Actions	Cues/prompts	Rationale based on Physiology
0–5 min	Includes: • Vital Signs • System-Specific Assessments • Verbal sounds	1. 2. 3. 4. 5.	1. 2. 3. 4. 5	(i.e., skin warm and moist related to febrile state, etc.)
5–10 min		1. 2. 3. 4. 5.	1. 2. 3. 4. 5.	
10–15 min		1. 2. 3. 4. 5.	1. 2. 3. 4. 5.	
15–30 min		1. 2. 3. 4. 5.	1. 2. 3. 4. 5.	

SCENARIO DESIGN TEMPLATE *(cont'd)*

Set–Up for Simulation for Client Care			
Simulator Setting/Environment	**Need**	**Setting/Environment**	**Need**
Medium Fidelity/Bed(s):		Critical Care	
High Fidelity/Bed(s):		Medical Surgical Unit	
Chester Chest		Clinic	
IV Arm Task Trainer		Home	
Central Line Task Trainer		Other	
Other			

Preparation of the Manikin			
Allergy Bracelet		___ Cold ___ Hot Pack for cool, clammy skin	
ID Bracelet		Cyanosis-Location	
Medical Alert Bracelet		Diabetic Extremity	
__Abdomen __Sound __Injection __Bladder		Diaphoresis–spray bottle	
Altered Pupils		Drain	
Blue Pad		Edema (unopened KY lubricant package can be placed under the skin of manikin)	
Body Fluids/Secretions:		Eye Glasses	
Cast		Foley Catheter:	
Chest Tube		Hair	
Clothing			

Equipment at Bedside/Bedside Table			
Bedpan/Urinal		Incentive Spirometer w/instructions	
Client Cell Phone Magazine		O₂ Delivery Device	
Dressing Change Supplies		___Pump: ___ IV ___ Enteral (see orders for rate)	
Emesis Basin & Contents		Thermometer (see client vital signs)	
Food		Water Pitcher/cup/straw & Kleenex	
Glucometer (see client vital signs)		Wheelchair	
Incentive Spirometer w/ instructions		Other	
O₂ Delivery Device		Suction Kits	
___Pump: ___ IV ___ Enteral (see orders for rate)		Other	

cont'd on next page

APPENDIX C

SCENARIO DESIGN TEMPLATE *(cont'd)*

Set–Up for Simulation for Client Care *(cont'd)*			
Equipment Supply Care	**Need**	**Equipment Supply Care**	**Need**
Dressing Change Supplies :		Pulse Ox	
Foley Catheters		TED Hose	
IV		Tracheostomy/Suction Kits	
IV SLN		Wound dressing/Band-Aid	
IV Fluid Reservoir Bag		Narcotic box	
Manikin Physiologic Cues		Saline	
Medication Cup		Sterile Q-tip	
Nasogastric Tube, Irrigation Syringe & pH tape		Tongue Blades	
Ostomy		Towel/Washcloths	
O$_2$ Delivery Device (see orders for rate)		Other	
Medication (see orders for specific meds)		**Chart**	
Eye drops		Client Information Face Sheet	
IV Fluids		Admission Orders	
IVPB		Physician Orders	
IVP in med drawer		MAR	
Inhaler		Diagnostic Information	
____IM ____ Subcutaneous		History & Physical	
____PO ____ Sublingual		Lab	
Transdermal patch		Intake & Output	
Other		Progress Sheet	
		Kardex	

Med Cart/Room	Need	Forms	Need	Simulation Roles/Name Tags	Need
Saline Flush, NS, Tubing		Nurse Report		Patient Care Tech/Nurses Assistant	
Other:		Focused Assessment		Primary Nurse (2-3 nurses, see faculty overview)	
		Communication		Medication Nurse/LPN	
		Correct Action		Resource Nurse	
		Policy Procedure Book		Treatment Nurse	
		Narcotic Sign Out Form		Quality Assurance Monitor	
		Other		Documenter (Recorder)	
				Observer	
				Family Member or Significant Other	
				Other	

EXAMPLE OF AN ORIGINAL SCENARIO PACKET: PEDIATRIC EMERGENCY RESPONSE

Pediatric Emergency Response Simulation Course Name: Pediatrics	
Faculty Overview of Simulation *(2 pages; not for distribution to students)*	
Concepts: • Prioritization of ABCs • Thermoregulation Management • Assessment/Management during Pediatric Code **Client Name:** Jaclyn Jordan	**Learning Objectives:** • Identify acute respiratory failure in a pediatric client. • Respond appropriately to respiratory failure using ABC approach. • Recognize common causes/assessment in infant respiratory failure (including fluid status, low temperature, and hypoglycemia). • Incorporate family-centered care in an emergent pediatric care situation.
Placement in the Curriculum	
Low Stakes: Use as a formative stand-alone simulation or in a multi-station clinical experience.	**High Stakes:** May use as a high-stakes simulation (Refer to Chapter 6, Appendix B, Grading Rubric Using Base Points) or as part of a multi-station high-stakes simulation (Refer to Chapter 6, Appendix D, Grading Rubric for Multi-Station Simulation). High-stakes simulation is not recommended as first or only simulation activity in a course. Early in semester, recommend using a low-stakes simulation activity involving practicing steps of an emergency response.
Psychomotor Skills: • Hand hygiene • Physical assessment, including vital signs • Infant CPR • Glucometer use • Temperature regulation strategies	**Cognitive Skills:** • Nursing Process • Prioritization of ABCs • Identification of Hypothermia • National Patient Safety Goals • Communication using SBAR

Brief Overview and Goals of Simulation for Faculty Preparation
Jaclyn Jordan is a 6-week-old female admitted 4 days ago due to poor feeding and diarrhea x 2 days. She was diagnosed with moderate dehydration and gastroenteritis. She continues to have loose stools with some blood-streaked diarrhea and intermittent fever. Past medical history includes a healthy pregnancy and birth. She currently has maintenance IV fluids into a peripheral IV in her right hand. Upon entering the client's room, the student nurse will find Jaclyn with cyanosis and the following VS: RR–0/min, HR–30 bpm, O$_2$ Sat–76%. The client is currently in respiratory failure due to hypothermia–the client was recently unwrapped for a significant period while staff obtained a new IV. This is compounded by acute illness stressors and mother keeping the infant less covered to "prevent fevers." The goal of the scenario is for the student to recognize the need for CPR, call for emergency assistance, and address causes of infant respiratory failure.
Student Configuration: For a standard pediatrics or capstone course, it is recommended students complete this simulation in groups of 2–3. Alternatively, start the simulation with 1–2 students and send in a third student as a charge nurse or nurse colleague to assist once Code Blue Jr. is called/assistance is requested.

cont'd on next page

EXAMPLE OF AN ORIGINAL SCENARIO PACKET
PEDIATRIC EMERGENCY RESPONSE *(cont'd)*

Student Pre-Simulation Work
Information and practice can be covered in earlier content and/or assigned readings.
Content: National Patient Safety Goals (2017), Nursing assessment and management of pediatric emergencies, appropriate vital sign ranges for infant, causes and preventive measures for acute distress in infants
Practice (past simulation or clinical experiences): Standard precautions, CPR technique, temperature management for infants, SBAR

Pre-briefing Time 15 min	Simulation Time 10–12 min	Debriefing Time 30–40 min
Pre-Briefing Topics: • Identify the National Patient Safety Goals and describe priority plans to meet each goal. • Discuss resources and protocols in health care facilities to manage pediatric emergencies. • Discuss proactive steps RNs can take to reduce/prevent pediatric emergencies in ill clients. **Orientation to Unit:** • Standard orientation to simulation suite and equipment		

VERBAL REPORT TO STUDENTS

- Facilitating instructor will provide verbal report from the outgoing nurse (on next page of packet) at the end of pre-briefing.
- Provide students with the client chart containing provider orders, diagnostic report, and MAR.
- After report, allow 5 minutes for the students to plan their approach to situation.

REPORT FROM OUTGOING NURSE

Medical Diagnoses: Moderate dehydration, Gastroenteritis

Recent Surgeries/Procedures: n/a

Co-morbidities: n/a

Jaclyn Jordan is a 6-week-old female admitted 4 days ago due to poor feeding and diarrhea X 2 days at home. No known allergies. She weighed 5.1 kg this morning, this is the same as the past 2 days. When she first came in, her weight was 4.7 kg. She got 2 fluid boluses when she was admitted.

She has been having loose stools with some a little blood-streaked diarrhea since she was admitted, but stools are decreasing. She has had intermittent fever; last fever was last night. She has had good wet diapers, 3 on my shift plus probably some more in the diapers with diarrhea.

Her past medical history includes a healthy pregnancy and birth. No other past illnesses.

She has D5 ½ NS with 5 mEq KCL/L running at 33 mL /hr into a peripheral IV in her right hand. We just got that IV an hour ago. It took a while to get a good vein but we got it in 2 sticks.

She is on regular diet as tolerated, taking in about 2 ounces per bottle right now, Mom says that is about half of her usual. No medications except her fluids and PRN acetaminophen if she has a fever.

Vital signs are ordered for every 4 hours, the last set was taken 2 hours ago. Temp–98.2°F, heart rate–109 bpm, respiratory rate–28/min, blood pressure–88/60. She is on a continuous pulse ox; it was 98 %, I think or it was when I left after the infant received IV. Her mom is in the room with her; dad was here early last night, and went home to take care of their other child.

EXAMPLE OF AN ORIGINAL SCENARIO PACKET
PEDIATRIC EMERGENCY RESPONSE *(cont'd)*

SIMULATION—CLIENT CARE				
Time (Estimated time only, go with student progression)	**Manikin Settings & Changes**	**Student Actions**	**Cues/ Prompts**	**Rationale Based on Physiology**

0–5 min	Set manikin as able; other findings may be verbalized via overhead speaker if students assess area:
	
	Vital Sign Initial Settings:
	
	HR: 30 bpm
	
	RR: 0/min
	
	O_2: 78%
	
	BP: 60/40
	
	Skin around mouth: blue/cyanotic
	
	Airway: clear
	
	Breath sounds: absent (set as clear on manikin for evaluations of rescue breathing)
	
	Cap refill: 3 seconds
	
	Pulses: +1 to 0
	
	Verbal sounds/movement: None
		1. Students identify client is in respiratory failure.
		
		2. *Actions:*
		
		  a. If students place oxygen via ambu bag around 20 or more breaths/minute, change manikin to: O_2 sats—88%, all other settings unchanged.
		
		  b. If students place oxygen via mask or provides ambu bag at < 20 breaths/minute, change manikin to: O_2 sats—70%, HR—20 bpm.
		
		  If students then change to ambu bag at appropriate rate, follow 2a: O_2 sats—88%, HR—30 bpm.
		
		  c. If students do not provide oxygen in any form within 2 minutes, change O_2 sats—50%, HR—15 bpm.
		
		  d. If students then place O_2, go with 2a or 2b above, based on oxygen delivery.
		
		  e. If students do not provide oxygen beyond 3 minutes, O_2 sats to "unreadable" or 0, HR to 0 bpm. If students then place O_2, go with 2a or 2b above, with slower rebound.
		
		  f. If students do not provide oxygen within 5 minutes, stop scenario.
			If student action is 2c (in low-stakes only):
			
			Consider having an instructor facilitator play the role of a supply tech and step in room to drop off IV fluid bag and say, "Looks like they need serious help!" This hopefully will prompt the student to see the infant is blue and not breathing.
				Skin around mouth is blue/cyanotic; cap refill 3 seconds; weak pulses; no movement, no sound, due to acute respiratory failure.
				
				RR is set at 0 rather than 5-10 as might be first seen in this situation to reduce student confusion and assist in moving towards appropriate action.

cont'd on next page

APPENDIX D

EXAMPLE OF AN ORIGINAL SCENARIO PACKET
PEDIATRIC EMERGENCY RESPONSE *(cont'd)*

SIMULATION–CLIENT CARE *(cont'd)*				
Time (Estimated time only, go with student progression)	**Manikin Settings & Changes**	**Student Actions**	**Cues/ Prompts**	**Rationale Based on Physiology**
5–9 min		After progress through 2a or 2b, students identify need for compressions. 3. *Actions:* a. If students providing 100 + compressions/minute, change to O_2 sat–95%, HR 60, turn off cyanosis. b. If students provide compressions at slower rate, change O_2 sat–90%, HR–45 bpm; If students increase compression rate, follow 3a. c. If students do not provide compressions within 4 minutes, change O_2 sat to 30%, HR–15 bpm; If students then provide compressions, go to 3a or 3b. d. If students do not provide compressions within additional 30 seconds, O_2 Sat 10%, HR–5 bpm. e. If student continues without compressions, stop scenario. f. If student initiates compressions, go to 3a or 3b as appropriate.	Follow steps and end scenario if students' progress through 3c.	Skin around mouth is blue/ cyanotic and may improve, related to nursing care provided during respiratory failure state.

EXAMPLE OF AN ORIGINAL SCENARIO PACKET
PEDIATRIC EMERGENCY RESPONSE *(cont'd)*

SIMULATION—CLIENT CARE *(cont'd)*				
Time (Estimated time only, go with student progression)	**Manikin Settings & Changes**	**Student Actions**	**Cues/ Prompts**	**Rationale Based on Physiology**

9–11 min	After CPR is fully initiated, vital signs modified based on student action (See second column for details). Settings for automated trending response to tasks:
	
	HR: 100 bpm (slow progression once compressions start)
	
	RR: 8/min
	
	BP: 70/50
	
	O$_2$: Sat 95%
	
	Cap refill 2 seconds
		1. Students call CODE BLUE JR. or Rapid Response within 2 minutes.
		
		2. Students reassess client and find sustained HR–100 bpm, RR–8/min.
		
		3. *Action:*
		
		  a. If students restart ambu bag, maintain VS changes as is. If students also restart compressions, maintain VS changes as is.
		
		  b. If students do not restart ambu bag within 1 minute of reassessment, change to HR–60 bpm, RR–0/min, BP–60/40, Sat–60%, and return cyanosis.
		
		  c. If students restart ambu bag, go to 6a.
		
		  d. If students do not restart ambu bag, change to HR–40 bpm, RR–0/min, O$_2$ Sat–40%, then end scenario.
			If no Code/ Rapid Response called within 4 minutes, parent should ask, "Shouldn't you get some help?"	HR improvement, weak pulse, cap refill 2 seconds, related to student actions with CPR.
				
				Code Blue or Code Blue Jr. is the accurate emergency response for the situation. A student may call a Rapid Response instead, which is not optimal recognition of situation but would bring expert assistance.
				
				Use ambu bag as needed anytime there are no/insufficient respirations.
				
				Chest compressions are not needed at this stage due to HR, but are not harmful.

cont'd on next page

APPENDIX D

EXAMPLE OF AN ORIGINAL SCENARIO PACKET
PEDIATRIC EMERGENCY RESPONSE *(cont'd)*

SIMULATION—CLIENT CARE *(cont'd)*				
Time (Estimated time only, go with student progression)	**Manikin Settings & Changes**	**Student Actions**	**Cues/ Prompts**	**Rationale Based on Physiology**
11–12 min		1. Students assess causes of infant respiratory failure to correct. 2. *Action*: a. If student assesses hydration status, report findings of any area consistent with sufficient hydration (such as no tenting of skin, mucous membranes moist). Cap refill is 2–3 seconds depending on O_2 sat. b. If students use glucometer, report result as 85 mg/dL. c. If students assess temperature, report result as 95.2°F (If they assess temperature in first 2 minutes of scenario, recommend reporting result as 95.5°F). 3. *Action:* a. If students turn on Radiant Heat Warmer and fully uncover infant or students apply a warm blanket and hat, facilitator should announce "10 minutes has passed," then change manikin to HR–105 bpm, RR–20/min, infant weakly fussing/crying, BP–70/50, O_2 sat–97%. **End Scenario.**	If students discuss potential for dehydration, parent should report changing diaper right after the new IV start that was "pretty wet." If students are not checking temperature after getting VS up to sustainable levels, parent can say, "I only put a blanket on her. I didn't want her to get another fever."	If action taken to correct temperature, client will return to more stable baseline.

EXAMPLE OF AN ORIGINAL SCENARIO PACKET
PEDIATRIC EMERGENCY RESPONSE *(cont'd)*

Provider Communication

- Students should contact provider to report infant's status.
- Students may appropriately contact provider at any point in the scenario. Facilitator should respond based ONLY on information provided in the SBAR report. It is important to use only the prompts provided to ensure the simulation is consistent from one time to the next and that each student receives the same information.
- If student reports respiratory failure but has not identified cause, provider should ask questions about wet diapers, temperature, and blood sugar; encourage student to continue to provide CPR as appropriate and call back if identify need for an order.
- Provider should not provide orders for any medications. If asked about epinephrine or other cardiac stimulants, respond for students to continue CPR, seek causes, and that Code team is on the way (if they have called them).
- In all situations, provider should report they are on the way to assist.

Set–Up for Simulation for Client Care			
Simulator Setting/Environment	**Need**	**Setting/Environment**	**Need**
Medium Fidelity/Bed(s):		Critical Care	
High Fidelity/Bed(s): X female infant	**X**	Medical Surgical Unit	
Chester Chest		Clinic	
IV Arm Task Trainer		Home	
Central Line Task Trainer		Other: **Pediatric Unit**	
Other			

Preparation of the Manikin			
Allergy Bracelet		___ Cold ___ Hot Pack for cool, clammy skin	
ID Bracelet	**X**	**Cyanosis–Location Lips, per manikin programming (or blue eye shadow on cellophane around mouth if low-fidelity)**	**X**
Medical Alert Bracelet		Diabetic Extremity	
__Abdomen __Sound __Injection __Bladder		Diaphoresis – spray bottle	
Altered Pupils		Drain	
Blue Pad		Edema (unopened KY lubricant package can be placed under the skin of manikin)	
Body Fluids/Secretions:		Eye Glasses	
Cast		Foley Catheter:	
Chest Tube		Hair	
Clothing: Only a diaper on infant with loose single blanket laid on top, infant hat and socks in bassinet.	**X**		

cont'd on next page

APPENDIX D

Chapter 5

EXAMPLE OF AN ORIGINAL SCENARIO PACKET
PEDIATRIC EMERGENCY RESPONSE *(cont'd)*

Equipment at Bedside/Bedside Table			
Bedpan/Urinal		Incentive Spirometer w/instructions	
Client Cell Phone Magazine		O₂ Delivery Device—Infant & Peds-sized ambu bags with masks & infant face mask	X
Dressing Change Supplies		_X_ Pump: _X_ IV ___ Enteral (see orders for rate)	X
Emesis Basin & Contents		Thermometer (see client vital signs)	
Food		Water Pitcher/cup/straw & Kleenex	
Glucometer (see client vital signs)		Wheelchair	
Incentive Spirometer w/ instructions		**Other: warming blankets**	X
O₂ Delivery Device		**Suction Kits—Nasal and Yankauer Suction Kits**	X
___Pump: ___ IV ___ Enteral (see orders for rate)		**Other—Thermometer & Blood Pressure Cuff**	X

Setup for Simulation for Client Care *(cont'd)*			
Equipment Supply Care	**Need**	**Equipment Supply Care**	**Need**
Dressing Change Supplies :		**Pulse Ox**	X
Foley Catheters		TED Hose	
IV		Tracheostomy/Suction Kits	
IV SLN		Wound dressing/Band-Aid	
IV Fluid Reservoir Bag		Narcotic box	
Manikin physiologic cues		Saline	
Medication Cup		Sterile Q-tip	
Nasogastric Tube, Irrigation Syringe & pH tape		Tongue Blades	
Ostomy		Towel/Washcloths	
O₂ Delivery Device (see orders for rate)		Other	
Medication (see orders for specific meds)		**Chart**	
Eye drops		Client Information Face Sheet	
IV Fluids—D5 ½ NS W/5mEq KCL/L @ 33 mL/hr. on a pump	X	**Admission Orders**	X
IVPB		**Physician Orders**	X
IVP in med drawer		**MAR**	X
Inhaler		**Diagnostic Information**	X
___IM ___ Subcutaneous		History & Physical	
_X_ PO Acetaminophen liquid __ Sublingual	X	**Lab**	X
Transdermal patch		Intake & Output	
Other		Progress Sheet	
		Kardex	

EXAMPLE OF AN ORIGINAL SCENARIO PACKET
PEDIATRIC EMERGENCY RESPONSE *(cont'd)*

Med Cart/Room	Need	Forms	Need	Simulation Roles/Name Tags	Need
Saline Flush, NS, Tubing	X	Nurse Report		Patient Care Tech/Nurses Assistant	
Other:		Focused Assessment		Primary Nurse (2-3 nurses, see faculty overview)	
		Communication		Medication Nurse/LPN	
		Correct Action		Resource Nurse	
		Policy Procedure Book		Treatment Nurse	
		Narcotic Sign Out Form		Quality Assurance Monitor	
		Other		Documenter (Recorder)	
				Observer	
				Family Member or Significant Other	
				Other—Parent (instructor facilitator or a separate student volunteer)	X

cont'd on next page

APPENDIX D

EXAMPLE OF AN ORIGINAL SCENARIO PACKET
PEDIATRIC EMERGENCY RESPONSE *(cont'd)*

Simulation Hospital Medical Order Sheet

Client: Jordan, Jaclyn   MR#0040

Date/Time	Orders
4 days prior to Sim.	Admit to pediatric floor
	VS: Q 2 hours X 6 hours, then Q 4 hours
	Continuous pulse ox
	Daily weights, strict I and O
	Allergies: NKDA
	Fluids: D5 ½ NS @ 33 cc/hr (add 5 mEq KCL/L after 1st wet diaper). Also, give 50 mL NS bolus (10 cc/kg) via IV X 1. If urine output after 4 hours is less than 50 mL, repeat bolus X 1.
	Acetaminophen 30 mg po Q 4 hours PRN fever greater than 100.8, call provider before giving
	Admission Labs: BMP, CBC w/ diff, stool culture X 1
	X-ray: Abdominal X-ray without contrast, then Barium enema abdominal X-ray (rule out perforation and intussusception)
	Diet: NPO until after X-rays complete. Then, offer 1 oz. Infalyte Q 3 hours. If tolerated without vomiting X 6 hours, increase to 2 oz. Infalyte Q 3 hours.
	Provider Signature:

Date/Time	Orders
3 days prior to Sim.	BMP, CBC every AM
	Diet: Advance to home formula, starting with 1 oz. Q 3 hours. If tolerated, increase to 2 oz., then ad lib.
	Continue fluids, VS, weights, I and O, and acetaminophen as ordered
	Provider Signature:

Date/Time	Orders
	Provider Signature:

Date/Time	Orders
	Provider Signature:

EXAMPLE OF AN ORIGINAL SCENARIO PACKET
PEDIATRIC EMERGENCY RESPONSE *(cont'd)*

LAB RESULTS AND DIAGNOSTIC FINDINGS

Client: Jordan, Jaclyn, MR# 0040

Most recent labs *(obtained this morning)*:

CBC:	RBC 4.6 million cells/µL
	WBC 10,400 cells/µL
	Platelets 166,000 cells/µL
	Hemoglobin 9.9 grams/dL
	Hematocrit 30.8%
BMP:	Sodium 137 mEq/L
	Chloride 98 mEq/L
	Glucose 82 mg/dL
	Calcium 9.1 mg/dL
	Potassium 3.7 mEq/L
	CO_2 21 mEq/L
	Blood Urea Nitrogen 13 mg/dL
	Serum Creatinine 0.8 mg/dL

Past results:

Stool culture *(obtained on admission, results finalized 2 days ago)*:
    Positive for leukocytes
    Negative for E. coli 0157:H7, C. diff

Abdominal X-ray without contrast *(summary of results, obtained day of admission)*:
    No signs of perforation or obstruction
    Gas present in loops of bowel

Abdominal X-ray with Barium enema *(summary of results, obtained day of admission)*:
    No signs of twisted or obstructed bowel. Intussusception not indicated.

---

cont'd on next page

APPENDIX D

Chapter 5

EXAMPLE OF AN ORIGINAL SCENARIO PACKET
PEDIATRIC EMERGENCY RESPONSE *(cont'd)*

MEDICATION ADMINISTRATION RECORD

Client: Jordan, Jaclyn   6 weeks old, DOB: _____   Allergies: NKDA

	0700-1459	1500-2259	2300-0659
D5 ½ NS w/ 5 mEq KCL/L @ 33 mL/hr			
Acetaminophen 30 mg PO Q 4 hours PRN fever greater than 100.8° F			

EXAMPLE OF AN ORIGINAL SCENARIO PACKET
PEDIATRIC EMERGENCY RESPONSE *(cont'd)*

SIMULATION DEBRIEF GUIDE POINTS: PEDIATRIC EMERGENCY RESPONSE

Follow the DML (Debrief for Meaningful Learning) process as discussed in Chapter 5 to promote a student-driven learning opportunity. Given the acute and high-stress nature of the simulated situation in this scenario, faculty guidance through emotional, mental, and skill-based concerns are critical.

Potential Areas to Incorporate or Highlight During Debrief:

Prioritization of Airway, Breathing and Circulation

- Recognize there are pediatric differences. The likelihood is increased in a pediatric emergency that the problem is due to respiratory causes. Respiratory intervention can be critical.

CPR Technique

- Based on performance in the simulation, review basic technique as needed.
  - o Ratio for 1 and 2 provider CPR.
  - o Rescue breath and compression skills.
  - o Use of ambu bag with oxygen at 10+ L pm to maximize benefit.
    Clarify purpose of 10 Liters O_2 with ambu bag (provides 100% oxygen flow in emergency compared to 10 Liters via a face mask).

- Review when to initiate rescue breathing (pediatric rule of thumb: when half of expected rate for age or insufficient effort).
  - o Ventilations support oxygenation—providing rescue breaths early may prevent worsening status and, depending on cause, may even prevent the need for compressions.

- Review when to initiate chest compressions (pediatric rule of thumb: when half of expected rate for age or unable to palpate a pulse).
  - o Compressions support perfusion—waiting until HR is absent makes it more difficult to rescue situation. Some pediatric situations will stabilize with minimal intervention.

Treatment and Prevention of Temperature Regulation Issues

- **Treatment options include:**
  - o Radiant Heat Warmer. Infant should be uncovered, temperature monitor in place on skin with alarm set for extremes, eye covering, and hourly checks of infant temperature.
  - o Warmed blankets, hat, socks.

- **Prevention measures include:**
  - o Keep infant as covered as possible during procedures.
  - o Check temperature after procedures, even if it is not time for routine check.

Family-Centered Care

- Discuss parent presence in pediatric emergencies, include the positive points and the drawbacks. Discuss how to update parent and get valuable input from parent. If parent prompts were needed in the simulation today, point out the value of this input.

APPENDIX E
Chapter 5

EXAMPLE OF AN ORIGINAL SCENARIO PACKET: ADULT RESPIRATORY DISTRESS DUE TO HYPOVOLEMIA

Adult Respiratory Distress Due to Hypovolemia Course Name: Adult Health I, II or Capstone	
Faculty Overview of Simulation *(2 pages; not for distribution to students)*	
Concepts: • Prioritization of ABCs • Assessment of Causes of Respiratory Distress • Management of Acute Adult Respiratory Distress **Client Name:** Robert Willis	**Learning Objectives:** • Identify acute respiratory failure in an adult client. • Respond appropriately to respiratory distress using ABC approach. • Recognize common causes/system specific assessments in respiratory distress (including fluid status, infection, and obstruction).
Placement in the Curriculum	
Low Stakes: Use as a formative stand-alone simulation or in a multi-station clinical experience.	**High Stakes:** May use as a high-stakes simulation (Refer to Chapter 6, Appendix B, Grading Rubric Using Base Points) or as part of a multi-station high-stakes simulation (Refer to Chapter 6, Appendix D, Grading Rubric for Multi-Station Simulation). High-stakes simulation is not recommended as first or only simulation activity in a course. Early in semester, recommend using a low-stakes simulation activity involving practicing steps of an emergency response.
Psychomotor Skills: • Hand hygiene • Physical assessment, including vital signs • Oxygen equipment application • IV fluid administration	**Cognitive Skills:** • Nursing Process • Prioritization of ABCs • Identification of Fluid Volume Deficit • National Patient Safety Goals • Communication using SBAR

Brief Overview and Goals of Simulation for Faculty Preparation
Robert Willis is a 46-year-old male in the ER complaining of being "really out of breath." He reports the shortness of breath started, "maybe a couple days ago" and says "it got worse today when I was working out at the gym" so he came to the ER. His friend at the gym drove him here on his way to work. Asked about any other symptoms or complaints recently, he reports, "nothing really, heartburn in the past few weeks with some dull pain sometimes in my stomach" and "I've been feeling sick to my stomach the past few days but I think that is from having trouble breathing." Past medical history is unremarkable except for asthma, when he was 6 or 7 years old. He has a peripheral IV in his right hand. Upon entering the client's room, the student nurse will find Robert sitting high in bed with the following VS: Temp–98.9°F, RR–27/min, HR–106 bpm, BP 118/70, O_2 Sat–86% on 2 L O_2 via nasal cannula. There is a small amount of acute blood/coffee ground-mixed emesis on the front of the client's shirt. The client is currently in respiratory distress due to hypovolemia from an unrecognized bleeding peptic ulcer. The goal of the scenario is for the student to recognize the signs of hypovolemia and assess further to address causes beyond respiratory issues, notify provider of client's condition, and address causes of acute respiratory distress.

Student Configuration:
For a standard medical-surgical or capstone course, it is recommended students complete this simulation in pairs or alone. Alternatively, start the simulation with one student and send in a second student as a charge nurse or nurse colleague to assist at a designated time point or progress point in the scenario.

EXAMPLE OF AN ORIGINAL SCENARIO PACKET:
ADULT RESPIRATORY DISTRESS DUE TO HYPOVOLEMIA *(cont'd)*

Student Pre-Simulation Work		
(Sections can be covered in course content or earlier clinicals; sections may be assigned via readings.)		
Pre-briefing Time 15 min	Simulation Time 10–12 min	Debriefing Time 30–40 min
Pre-Briefing Topics: • Identify the National Patient Safety Goals (2017), and describe priority plans to meet each goal. • Discuss focused assessment for a specific symptom, then considering assessments of potential causes for a specific symptom. • Discuss steps of SBAR and updating provider on status changes in acute care settings. **Orientation to Unit:** • Standard orientation to simulation suite and equipment		

VERBAL REPORT TO STUDENTS

- Facilitating instructor will provide verbal report from the outgoing nurse (on next page of packet) at the end of pre-briefing.

- Provide students with the client chart containing provider orders, diagnostic report, and MAR.

- After report, allow 5 minutes for the students to plan their approach to situation.

REPORT FROM OUTGOING NURSE

Medical Diagnoses: Shortness of Breath

Recent Surgeries/Procedures: n/a

Co-morbidities: n/a

Robert Willis is a 46-year-old male who came to the ER complaining of being "really out of breath" two and a half hours ago. He reported the shortness of breath starting "maybe a couple days ago" and says "it got worse today when I was working out at the gym" so he came to the ER. His friend from the gym drove him here on his way to work. I asked him about any other symptoms or complaints recently, he said, "Nothing really, heartburn in the past few weeks with some dull pain sometimes in my stomach" and "feeling sick to my stomach past few days but I think that is from having trouble breathing." Past medical history is unremarkable except for asthma, when he was 6 or 7 years old. His weight is 79 kg.

He has a peripheral IV in his right hand. I started it an hour ago and got the labs, haven't checked them yet in the computer.

He has no known allergies and doesn't take any home medications. We gave him 1 Albuterol treatment about two hours ago, in case he is having an asthma attack. His lungs sounded clear but I think the healthcare provider is making sure since he hasn't ever had any other breathing problems except for when he was a kid. It didn't really change any of his assessments, saturation stayed the same. It is ordered PRN q 2 hours if you think he needs it.

Vital signs are ordered hourly with continuous pulse oximetry. His last vital signs were an hour ago so the next set is due. Last vital signs were: Temp–98.8°F, RR–25/min, HR–102 bpm, BP–120/76, O_2 Sat–89% on 1/L O_2 via nasal cannula. The orders say to keep O_2 above 90% so I increased the oxygen to 2 liters.

cont'd on next page

APPENDIX E

EXAMPLE OF AN ORIGINAL SCENARIO PACKET:
ADULT RESPIRATORY DISTRESS DUE TO HYPOVOLEMIA *(cont'd)*

SIMULATION—CLIENT CARE				
Time (Estimated time only, go with student progression)	**Manikin Settings & Changes**	**Student Actions**	**Cues/ Prompts**	**Rationale Based on Physiology**
0–5 min	Set manikin as able; other findings may be verbalized via overhead speaker if students assess area: **Vital Sign Initial Settings:** HR: 106 bpm RR: 27/min O$_2$: 86% with 2/L Oxygen via NC BP: 110/70 Airway: clear Breath sounds: clear Cap refill: 3 seconds Pulses: +2 Verbal sounds/ movement: manikin is sitting with HOB very elevated. Responds to questions with short answers and sounds breathless.	1. Students assess respiratory status. 2. *Actions:* a. If students increase oxygen via NC, change manikin to: O$_2$ sats–89%, all other settings unchanged. b. If students place oxygen via face mask at 5/L O$_2$ or more, change manikin to: O$_2$ sats–92%, all other settings unchanged. c. If students place oxygen via face mask at less than 5/L O$_2$, change manikin to: O$_2$ sats–84%, all other settings unchanged. d. If students do not increase oxygen delivery within first 3 minutes, decrease O$_2$ sats to 82%, increase RR to 30/min. e. If students then increase O$_2$, go with 2a, 2b, or 2c above. f. If students do not increase oxygen delivery within 8 minutes, decrease O$_2$ sats, down to 80%, increase RR to 33/min and increase HR to 116 bpm. g. If students then increase O$_2$, go with 2a, 2b, or 2c above. h. If students do not increase oxygen delivery but provide a dose of Albuterol, O$_2$ sats should remain unchanged/go along with increased oxygen as above if simultaneous, increase HR to 120 bpm.		Elevated RR and HR, with lower BP and oxygen saturation are caused by hypovolemia from a bleeding peptic ulcer.

EXAMPLE OF AN ORIGINAL SCENARIO PACKET:
ADULT RESPIRATORY DISTRESS DUE TO HYPOVOLEMIA *(cont'd)*

| SIMULATION—CLIENT CARE *(cont'd)*			
Time (Estimated time only, go with student progression)	**Manikin Settings & Changes**	**Student Actions**	**Cues/ Prompts**	**Rationale Based on Physiology**
5–10 min		3. Students gather additional assessment information. 4. ***Actions:*** a. Students request lab results. b. Students asks client questions to obtain additional information. 1. Did you throw up? What color was it? 2. Is this the first time? 3. Have you had any changes in your bowel movements?	Manikin voice responses to questions should sound short of breath: 1. Yes, just now. 2. Yes, it looks really weird. 3. Ummm (thinking)… past few days, guess have been sort of weird looking? And dark?	Labs on request options: a. Loaded for viewing or monitoring. b. A facilitator brings in the lab result page. c. Students are instructed to call lab for results. (Be sure students are aware of procedure to obtain labs as part of the orientation.)

cont'd on next page

APPENDIX E

EXAMPLE OF AN ORIGINAL SCENARIO PACKET:
ADULT RESPIRATORY DISTRESS DUE TO HYPOVOLEMIA *(cont'd)*

\multicolumn{5}{SIMULATION—CLIENT CARE *(cont'd)*}
Time (Estimated time only, go with student progression)	**Manikin Settings & Changes**	**Student Actions**	**Cues/Prompts**	**Rationale Based on Physiology**
5–10 min		Students notify provider of lab results and assessment updates using SBAR. 5. *Actions:* a. If students provide abnormal lab values, new assessment findings related to GI, and VS update:	a. "Sounds like this could be a GI bleed and some dehydration…" *Orders to give:* Start D5 ½ NS @ 100 mL/hr, Give a 500 mL NS bolus. Make NPO, D/C Albuterol, Obtain Upper Endoscopy. "I am on my way to admit the client to the floor."	If the full set of findings is available, a conclusion related to GI bleeding leading to hypovolemia, and thus respiratory distress follows the client history and pathophysiology of these diagnoses.
		b. If students provide abnormal lab values and new assessment findings related to GI without VS update:	b. Same response as 5a. Then, request they obtain new VS and call back.	
		c. If students provide abnormal lab values and VS update without new GI findings:	c. "Sounds like some dehydration? Is there anything else going on?" *Orders to give:* Start D5 ½ NS @ 100 mL/hr. Give a 500 mL NS bolus.	
		d. If students provide new GI findings and VS update without lab values: e. If student does not notify provider within 8 minutes (for low-stakes only), manikin can make a comment of "are there any updates from my doctor?"	d. Same response as 5a. Then, ask "Do we have those lab results back yet?"	

EXAMPLE OF AN ORIGINAL SCENARIO PACKET:
ADULT RESPIRATORY DISTRESS DUE TO HYPOVOLEMIA *(cont'd)*

SIMULATION—CLIENT CARE *(cont'd)*				
Time (Estimated time only, go with student progression)	**Manikin Settings & Changes**	**Student Actions**	**Cues/Prompts**	**Rationale Based on Physiology**
10–15 min		6. Students initiate IV fluid treatment. 7. ***Actions:*** a. If starts both maintenance fluids and accompanying bolus, announce overhead "Bolus is complete" and change VS to: O_2 sats, up to 92% if not already there due to oxygen in Steps 1 & 2; decrease RR to 23/min, decrease HR to 100 bpm, and increase BP to 122/76. b. If starts only maintenance fluids, O_2 sats, up to 90% if not already there due to oxygen in Steps 1 & 2. c. If starts only the fluid bolus, announce overhead "Bolus is complete" and change VS to: O_2 sats, up to 92% if not already there due to oxygen in Steps 1 & 2; decrease RR to 23/min, decrease HR to 100 bpm, and increase BP to 122/76. **End Scenario**		If action taken to improve hydration status, client will return to more stable status while awaiting further evaluation and treatment.

cont'd on next page

APPENDIX E

EXAMPLE OF AN ORIGINAL SCENARIO PACKET:
ADULT RESPIRATORY DISTRESS DUE TO HYPOVOLEMIA *(cont'd)*

SIMULATION—CLIENT CARE *(cont'd)*

Provider Communication

- Students should contact provider to report abnormal lab results, new gastrointestinal (GI) findings, and vital sign changes/oxygen needs.

- Students may appropriately contact provider at any point in the scenario. Facilitator should respond based only on information provided in the SBAR report.

- If student reports worsening respiratory distress but has not identified cause, provider should ask questions about lab results and other assessments, and call back if identify need for an order.

- Provider should not provide orders for any medications other than what is indicated in the chart above. If asked about other possibilities, respond that you will consider whether this is part of best plan.

SETUP FOR SIMULATION—CLIENT CARE

SetUp for Simulation for Client Care			
Simulator Setting/Environment	**Need**	**Setting/Environment**	**Need**
Medium Fidelity/Bed(s):		Critical Care	
High Fidelity/Bed(s): _X_ male	X	Medical Surgical Unit	
Chester Chest		Clinic	
IV Arm Task Trainer		Home	
Central Line Task Trainer		Other: **ER**	X
Other			

Preparation of the Manikin			
Allergy Bracelet		___ Cold ___ Hot Pack for cool, clammy skin	
ID Bracelet	X	Cyanosis—Location	
Medical Alert Bracelet		Diabetic Extremity	
__Abdomen __Sound __Injection __Bladder		Diaphoresis—spray bottle	
Altered Pupils		Drain	
Blue Pad		Edema (unopened KY lubricant package can be placed under the skin of manikin)	
Body Fluids/Secretions: simulated acute blood/coffee ground-mixed emesis (small amount on t-shirt, below)	X	Eye Glasses	
Cast		Foley Catheter	
Chest Tube		Hair	
Clothing: gym clothes (shorts, t-shirt)	X		

EXAMPLE OF AN ORIGINAL SCENARIO PACKET:
ADULT RESPIRATORY DISTRESS DUE TO HYPOVOLEMIA *(cont'd)*

Equipment at Bedside/Bedside Table			
Equipment Supply Care	**Need**	**Equipment Supply Care**	**Need**
Bedpan/Urinal		Incentive Spirometer w/instructions	
Client Cell Phone Magazine		**O₂ Delivery Device—Adult-sized Ambu-bag with mask & adult nasal cannula (on client), face mask, NRB mask**	**X**
Dressing Change Supplies		**_X_ Pump: _X_ IV** ____ Enteral (see orders for rate)	**X**
Emesis Basin & Contents		Thermometer (see client vital signs)	**X**
Food		Water Pitcher/cup/straw & Kleenex	
Glucometer (see client vital signs)		Wheelchair	
Incentive Spirometer w/ instructions		Other	
O₂ Delivery Device		**Suction Kits—NET and Yankauer Suction Kits**	**X**
___Pump: ___ IV ___ Enteral (see orders for rate)		**Other—Blood Pressure Cuff**	**X**

Equipment Supply Care	**Need**	**Equipment Supply Care**	**Need**
Dressing Change Supplies :		**Pulse Ox**	**X**
Foley Catheters		TED Hose	
IV		Tracheostomy/Suction Kits	
IV SLN		Wound dressing/Band-Aid	
IV Fluid Reservoir Bag		Narcotic box	
Manikin physiologic cues		Saline	
Medication Cup		Sterile Q-tip	
Nasogastric Tube, Irrigation Syringe & pH tape		Tongue Blades	
Ostomy		Towel/Washcloths	
O₂ Delivery Device (see orders for rate)		Other	
Medication (see orders for specific meds)		**Chart**	
Eye drops		Client Information Face Sheet	
IV Fluids in med drawer (D5 ½ NS)	**X**	**Admission Orders**	**X**
IVPB		**Physician Orders**	**X**
IVP in med drawer		**MAR**	**X**
Inhaler—Albuterol	**X**	**Diagnostic Information**	**X**
___IM ___Subcutaneous		History & Physical	
___PO ___Sublingual		**Lab**	**X**
Transdermal patch		Intake & Output	
Other		Progress Sheet	
		Kardex	

cont'd on next page

APPENDIX E

Chapter 5

EXAMPLE OF AN ORIGINAL SCENARIO PACKET:
ADULT RESPIRATORY DISTRESS DUE TO HYPOVOLEMIA *(cont'd)*

SETUP FOR SIMULATION—CLIENT CARE *(cont'd)*

Med Cart/Room	Need	Forms	Need	Simulation Roles/Name Tags	Need
Saline Flush, NS, Tubing	**X**	Nurse Report		Patient Care Tech/Nurses Assistant	
Other:		Focused Assessment		Primary Nurse **(1–2, see faculty overview)**	**X**
		Communication		Medication Nurse/LPN	
		Correct Action		Resource Nurse	
		Policy Procedure Book		Treatment Nurse	
		Narcotic Sign Out Form		Quality Assurance Monitor	
		Other		Documenter (Recorder)	
				Observer	
				Other	

EXAMPLE OF AN ORIGINAL SCENARIO PACKET:
ADULT RESPIRATORY DISTRESS DUE TO HYPOVOLEMIA *(cont'd)*

SIMULATION HOSPITAL MEDICAL ORDER SHEET

Client: Willis, Robert MR #0041

Date/Time	Orders
(2½ hours ago)	VS: Hourly
	Continuous pulse ox, apply O_2 via nasal cannula to keep sats > 90%
	Meds: Albuterol MDI 2 puffs Q 2 hours PRN wheezing, asthma symptoms
	Allergies: NKDA
	Labs: BMP, CBC
	Diet: Clear liquids. Advance as tolerated per respiratory effort.
	Provider Signature:

Date/Time	Orders
	Provider Signature:

Date/Time	Orders
	Provider Signature:

Date/Time	Orders
	Provider Signature:

cont'd on next page

APPENDIX E

EXAMPLE OF AN ORIGINAL SCENARIO PACKET:
ADULT RESPIRATORY DISTRESS DUE TO HYPOVOLEMIA *(cont'd)*

LAB RESULTS AND DIAGNOSTIC FINDINGS

Client: Willis, Robert MR #0041

Most recent labs *(obtained this morning):*

CBC:

RBC: 4.1 million cells/μL

WBC: 4,900 cells/μL

Platelets: 136,000 cells/μL

Hemoglobin: 9.7 grams/dL

Hematocrit: 34.8%

BMP:

Sodium: 148 mEq/L

Chloride: 98 mEq/L

Glucose: 105 mg/dL

Calcium: 9.1 mg/dL

Potassium: 4.4mEq/L

CO_2: 22 mEq/L

Blood Urea Nitrogen: 20 mg/dL

Serum Creatinine: 1.2 mg/dL

Serum Osmolality: 298 mOsm/kg

EXAMPLE OF AN ORIGINAL SCENARIO PACKET:
ADULT RESPIRATORY DISTRESS DUE TO HYPOVOLEMIA *(cont'd)*

MEDICATION ADMINISTRATION RECORD

Client: Willis, Robert   42 years old, DOB: _____   Allergies: NKDA

	0700-1459	1500-2259	2300-0659
Albuterol MDI 2 puffs Q 2 hours PRN wheezing, asthma symptoms			

cont'd on next page

EXAMPLE OF AN ORIGINAL SCENARIO PACKET:
ADULT RESPIRATORY DISTRESS DUE TO HYPOVOLEMIA *(cont'd)*

SIMULATION DEBRIEF GUIDE POINTS: ACUTE RESPIRATORY DISTRESS

Follow the DML (Debrief for Meaningful Learning) process as discussed in Chapter 5 to promote a student-driven learning opportunity.

Potential Areas to Incorporate or Highlight During Debrief:

Prioritization of Airway, Breathing and Circulation
- Recognizing vital sign trending. Discuss the pattern of each vital sign and what these collectively suggest is occurring (even noting that temperature is going down as body is less able to maintain temperature because of worsening hypovolemia).
- Recognizing other signs of respiratory distress (positioning in highest sitting position, short verbal responses).

Recognizing Potential Causes of Respiratory Distress and Assessing to Find Cause(s)
- Differentiation of Respiratory and Other System Causes based on VS patterns, breath sounds, intake/output, system-specific findings (i.e., increase in lab values, blood in emesis, unilateral changes in neurologic responses, cardiac dysrhythmias, etc.).
  - o Upper Respiratory Obstruction (airway swelling)
  - o Lower Respiratory Obstruction (asthma, spasms)
  - o Hypovolemia
  - o Brain Injury or Illness
  - o Cardiac Dysfunction (Myocardial Infarction, Heart Failure)

Oxygen Delivery Devices
- Amount of oxygen effectively used with each device; situations where each is useful or may be less desired means.
  - o Nasal cannula
  - o Face mask
  - o Non-rebreather mask
  - o Ambu bag
- Safety
  - o Fire prevention (no smoking or other flames; no petroleum-based lubricants)
  - o Equipment fit for true delivery
  - o Need for functioning oxygen (especially with masks, if loss of power driving oxygen system in facility, need to change to tanks emergently to avoid cutting off air flow to clients)

Treatment of Hypovolemia
- Maintenance fluids to provide baseline support compared to boluses to rapidly replace the fluid loss.
  - o Boluses should be given with isotonic fluids in almost all situations to reduce the risk of cerebral edema and avoid unnecessary blood sugar or other cellular shifts (NS, LR)
  - o Avoid bolusing directly from maintenance fluids
  - o In an evolving vital signs or LOC situation, the fluid bolus is high priority

SCREENSHOT OF ONLINE ORIENTATION COURSE

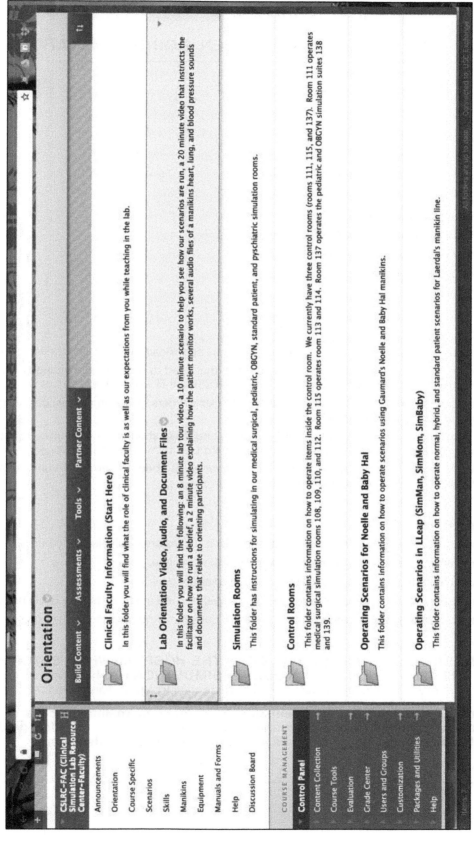

CSLRC-FAC (Clinical Simulation Lab Resource Center-Faculty)

Announcements
Orientation
Course Specific
Scenarios
Skills
Manikins
Equipment
Manuals and Forms
Help
Discussion Board

COURSE MANAGEMENT

Control Panel
Content Collection
Course Tools
Evaluation
Grade Center
Users and Groups
Customization
Packages and Utilities
Help

Orientation

Build Content ∨   Assessments ∨   Tools ∨   Partner Content ∨

Clinical Faculty Information (Start Here)
In this folder you will find what the role of clinical faculty is as well as our expectations from you while teaching in the lab.

Lab Orientation Video, Audio, and Document Files
In this folder you will find the following: an 8 minute lab tour video, a 10 minute scenario to help you see how our scenarios are run, a 20 minute video that instructs the facilitator on how to run a debrief, a 2 minute video explaining how the patient monitor works, several audio files of a manikins heart, lung, and blood pressure sounds and documents that relate to orienting participants.

Simulation Rooms
This folder has instructions for simulating in our medical surgical, pediatric, OBGYN, standard patient, and pyschiatric simulation rooms.

Control Rooms
This folder contains information on how to operate items inside the control room. We currently have three control rooms (rooms 111, 115, and 137). Room 111 operates medical surgical simulation rooms 108, 109, 110, and 112. Room 115 operates room 113 and 114. Room 137 operates the pediatric and OBGYN simulation suites 138 and 139.

Operating Scenarios for Noelle and Baby Hal
This folder contains information on how to operate scenarios using Gaumard's Noelle and Baby Hal manikins.

Operating Scenarios in LLeap (SimMan, SimMom, SimBaby)
This folder contains information on how to operate normal, hybrid, and standard patient scenarios for Laerdal's manikin line.

125

APPENDIX G

HELPFUL TIPS WHEN DOING SIMULATION

Required Equipment
- Stethoscope
- Penlight
- Scissors
- Pen/paper (clipboard)
- Watch with second hand

Professional Appearance
- Hair in compliance with clinical dress code
- Proper uniform with name tag
- Nails clean and short
- Minimal jewelry

Teamwork
- Work as a team-no one person is in charge unless specifically assigned by the faculty member.
- Prior to starting the scenario divide up activities that need to be done and change around from week to week (i.e., if student A does vital signs one week student B will do them the next).
- Each student should actively participate i.e. checking orders, preparing meds, checking IV site and fluids, communicating with the client, etc.
- All assessments, observations, communications and tasks should be communicated **out loud** to facilitate group decision making and give faculty insight into your thinking/planning process.
- If you feel you are on the right track or another student is about to perform an unsafe/inappropriate action, don't back down! Talk it out with your team.

Functional Points
- Healthcare Provider (HCP) orders and medication record are available at the bedside.
- Know where the supplies needed are kept for the scenario.
- Know the method for calling the HCP or other ancillary personnel.
- Lab results will be made available only if requested. If none are available the facilitator will state as much.
- **Treat the manikin as a real client** ... ask them questions and respond to their comments and questions.

REMEMBER THAT ACTIVITIES YOU DO IN THE HOSPITAL WHEN ENTERING THE CLIENT'S ROOM ARE ALSO EXPECTATIONS DURING SIMULATION (i.e., handwashing, identifying self using first and last name and your role as an RN, and identifying client using two identifiers).

Remember you signed a Confidentiality Agreement to maintain scenario integrity. Sharing information devalues student experiences, skews evaluation and/or grading expectations against earlier teams, and decreases learning experience for later teams.

TEMPLATE FOR SCHEDULING SIMULATION AND SKILL STATIONS

Time	Group A	Group B	Group C
0800–0830	Preconference	Preconference	Preconference
0830–0930	Scenario 1	Scenario 2	Skill Station
0930–1030	Scenario 3	Scenario 4	Scenario 1
1030–1130	Scenario 2	Scenario 3	Scenario 4
1130–1215	Lunch	Lunch	Lunch
1215–1315	Scenario 1	Scenario 2	Skill Station
1315–1415	Skill Station	Scenario 3	Scenario 4
1415–1515	Scenario 4	Skill Station	Scenario 3
1515–1600	Post-Conference	Post-Conference	Post-Conference

Developed by Kimberly Glenn, MN, RN, CNP

APPENDIX I

EXAMPLE OF CLINICAL DAY SIMULATION AND SKILL STATION SCHEDULE

Time	Group A	Group B	Group C
0800–0830	**Preconference** (Instructor A)	**Preconference** (Instructor B)	**Preconference** (Instructor C)
0830–0930	**Simulation:** Client Christine Jones with Bowel Resection/Colostomy	**Simulation:** Client Marilyn Hughes with Compartment Syndrome	**Skill Station: Colostomy care**
0930–1030	**Simulation:** Client Marilyn Hughes with Compartment Syndrome	**Skill Station: Colostomy care**	**Simulation:** Client Christine Jones with Bowel Resection/Colostomy
1030–1130	**Skill Station: Colostomy care**	**Simulation:** Client Christine Jones with Bowel Resection/Colostomy	**Simulation:** Client Marilyn Hughes with Compartment Syndrome
1130–1215	Lunch	Lunch	Lunch
1215–1315	**Station: Wound care**	**Activity:** Electronic Health Record–Document on Marilyn Hughes	**Simulation:** Client Christine Jones with Bowel Resection/Colostomy
1315–1415	**Simulation:** Client Christine Jones with Bowel Resection/Colostomy	**Station: Wound care**	**Activity:** Electronic Health Record–Document on Marilyn Hughes
1415–1515	**Activity:** Electronic Health Record–Document on Marilyn Hughes	**Simulation:** Client Christine Jones with Bowel Resection/Colostomy	**Station: Wound care**
1515–1600	**Post-Conference**	**Post-Conference**	**Post-Conference**

Colostomy Care:

Setup: 4 manikins with colostomies, all colostomy supplies at bedside.

Goal: Each student will select proper equipment, remove used appliance (filled with artificial stool) and apply new appliance.

Documentation: Procedure, stoma condition, client response, teaching.

Wound Care:

Setup: 4 manikins with open wound picture laminated onto their abdomen. Wound is covered with a serosanguinous dressing.

Goal: Each student will select proper equipment, remove old dressing properly and apply new dressing over the site.

Documentation: Procedure, wound condition, client response, teaching.

Activity:

Enter documentation from the Marilyn Hughes simulation experience into an electronic health record template.

TEMPLATE FOR SIMULATION LAB SETUP

Scenario/Skill	Skill Station Room	Scenario Room	Join Room	Debrief Room	Team Member In Control Room Y or N	Wired Student	Faculty Role/ Notes
IV Pump Review	105	N/A	N/A	N/A	N/A	N/A	*Faculty Member*
Marilyn Hughes w/Compartment Syndrome #1 & #2	N/A	108	113	113	Yes, Team Member 1	Yes–Friend #1 Family #2	*Neck Collar L arm splint Foley IV*
Christine Jones w/Bowel Resection & Colostomy #1 & #2	N/A	110	114	114	Yes, Team Member 2	Yes–Girlfriend	*Foley NG IV Abd Dsg/Drain*
EMR Review and Charting Exercise	105	N/A	N/A	N/A	N/A	N/A	*Faculty Member*

129

APPENDIX K

Chapter 5

EXAMPLE OF FACULTY SIMULATION GUIDE

Date: _____ Group #:_____

Faculty Guide for Evaluation

Use this form to create detailed evaluation information for your students. You can use this information in debriefing to quickly compare groups and also to help guide weekly evaluations. For the following, enter the information that you need in order to effectively evaluate the students in the simulation group.

Overall Scenario	
Did all group members wash their hands?	○ yes ○ no
Did all group members introduce themselves (first *and* last name, RN)?	○ yes ○ no
Was the client identified (name, DOB, read armband)?	○ yes ○ no
Vital Signs: Temp, Pulse, Respirations, BP & Other Vital Signs	T:____ P:____ R:____ BP:_____/_____ O$_2$ sat_____ Pain: ○ yes ○ no
What was included in the focused assessment (note if IV site and fluids were assessed)?	
Did students request labs?	○ yes ○ no
What was the interpretation of the lab results?	
Did students call the healthcare provider?	○ yes ○ no
What was included in SBAR?	
Was SBAR complete?	○ yes ○ no
Did the student write down and repeat back verbal orders?	○ yes ○ no

Individual			
	Name	Name	Name
Dress Code			
Participation			
Preparation			
Positive and Professional			
Teamwork/Communication			

Student Learning Objectives	
Recognize signs and symptoms of dehydration from their assessment.	○ Met ○ Not Met
Recognize relevant lab data associated with fluid imbalance.	○ Met ○ Not Met
Implement treatment of dehydration in a timely manner.	○ Met ○ Not Met
Implement and maintain client safety measures.	○ Met ○ Not Met
Implement communication with the multidisciplinary team members.	○ Met ○ Not Met

Developed by Cristy DeGregory PhD, RN

** *You may use back of form for additional comments.*

SIMULATION OBSERVER'S WORKSHEET

Student _____   Date _____

Learning Objectives:

1.

2.

3.

4.

ASSESSMENT (findings requiring action)	**ACTION** (action required by nurse)
TEAMWORK (collaborative actions)	**CLINICAL REASONING** (rationale for clinical or teamwork actions)

APPENDIX M

Chapter 5

WORKSHEET FOR DEBRIEFING FOR MEANINGFUL LEARNING (DML)

How did you feel about the simulation?	What went well during the simulation?	What would you do differently?

Dreifuerst, K. T. (2009)

CONSENT FOR SIMULATION LAB

Confidentiality Agreement

And

Authorization Release to be Videotaped

Course Name_____Date_____

Name_____

Telephone_____ Email_____

Location of Training_____

I understand and agree that I will not compromise or undermine the goals of the Clinical Simulation Laboratory (CSL). I further understand that discussions outside the training sessions may greatly diminish the effectiveness of the training and subject individuals to unwarranted criticism.

By signing below, I agree to maintain the strictest confidentiality regarding all observations of an individual's performance. I also agree not to discuss the content of any simulated training exercises outside of the CSL. Any breach of this contract will be reported to the Department Chairman or other appropriate authority and could result in disciplinary action against me.

By signing below, I also authorize CSL to photograph and/or record (video or audio) my training experience. I understand that any photograph and/or recordings resulting from this training session will be used solely for educational purposes, unless I give explicit authorization for them to be used for other purposes.

Print Your Name: _____

Participant Signature: _____

Date: _____

APPENDIX O

SIMULATION EXPERIENCE SURVEY FOR STUDENTS

	Strongly Disagree	Disagree	No Opinion	Agree	Strongly Agree	Not Applicable
1. The simulation-based scenario was appropriate for my level of learning.	1	2	3	4	5	6
2. The experience was appropriately placed in the overall curriculum.	1	2	3	4	5	6
3. The objectives of the simulation activity were clearly stated.	1	2	3	4	5	6
4. The scenario was a more effective learning experience compared to validating critical thinking in a clinical setting.	1	2	3	4	5	6
5. The course faculty and simulation staff provided me with important information to enhance my performance in the scenarios prior to and at the beginning of class.	1	2	3	4	5	6
6. The length of the total simulation/skill experience was adequate.	1	2	3	4	5	6
7. After completing the scenario, I felt better prepared to prioritize clients correctly.	1	2	3	4	5	6
8. After completing the scenario, I felt better prepared to intervene with my client's changing clinical status based on my assessments.	1	2	3	4	5	6
9. The simulation lab staff and scenario facilitators helped the check-off process to run smoothly.	1	2	3	4	5	6
10. I was prepared through clinical and coursework to handle the acuity level of the client(s) in the scenario.	1	2	3	4	5	6
11. I was prepared through clinical and coursework to process the detail of the client reports read before the scenario in the time that was provided.	1	2	3	4	5	6
12. The medication scenario and check off was appropriate for my level of learning.	1	2	3	4	5	6
13. The documentation case study was appropriate for my level of learning.	1	2	3	4	5	6
14. The debrief information helped me evaluate my own performance and improved my ability to prioritize.	1	2	3	4	5	6
15. The debrief assisted in my learning process and reinforced points of knowledge that I can apply to my practice in the clinical setting and improved by critical thinking.	1	2	3	4	5	6
16. The simulation experiences improved my knowledge on the classroom subjects/concepts covered.	1	2	3	4	5	6
17. I feel more confident in recognizing physiological changes in my clinical patients.	1	2	3	4	5	6
18. I feel more confident in my ability to communicate using the SBAR technique.	1	2	3	4	5	6

SIMULATION EXPERIENCE SURVEY FOR STUDENTS *(cont'd)*

19. What major aspects of the scenarios need improvement in order to achieve maximum realism?

20. If you could change one thing about this experience, what would it be?

21. If you could keep one thing about this experience the same, what would it be?

22. We value any comments about the scenario and any other aspect of your experience.

APPENDIX P

Faculty Simulation Orientation Evaluation

Please complete the following evaluation form to contribute information for future orientation classes on simulation. Feel free to be totally candid.

1. This class oriented me to the basic terms and definitions used in simulation.
   A. Strongly agree   B. Agree   C. Undecided   D. Disagree   E. Strongly Disagree

2. This class made me familiar with the capabilities of the high fidelity manikins.
   A. Strongly agree   B. Agree   C. Undecided   D. Disagree   E. Strongly Disagree

3. This class made me feel more knowledgeable about the process of running a simulation.
   A. Strongly agree   B. Agree   C. Undecided   D. Disagree   E. Strongly Disagree

4. I understand (with the help of an information sheet if necessary) how to start the scenario.
   A. Strongly agree   B. Agree   C. Undecided   D. Disagree   E. Strongly Disagree

5. I understand how to stop the scenario.
   A. Strongly agree   B. Agree   C. Undecided   D. Disagree   E. Strongly Disagree

6. I understand how to adjust vital signs on the manikin and change the waveform choice.
   A. Strongly agree   B. Agree   C. Undecided   D. Disagree   E. Strongly Disagree

7. I know how to adjust heart sounds, breath sounds and bowel sounds when needed.
   A. Strongly agree   B. Agree   C. Undecided   D. Disagree   E. Strongly Disagree

8. I know how to turn off the audible beep on the cardiac monitor.
   A. Strongly agree   B. Agree   C. Undecided   D. Disagree   E. Strongly Disagree

9. I understand the purpose of debriefing.
   A. Strongly agree   B. Agree   C. Undecided   D. Disagree   E. Strongly Disagree

10. I feel that using the debrief worksheet will help me organize the debrief sessions I run.
    A. Strongly agree   B. Agree   C. Undecided   D. Disagree   E. Strongly Disagree

11. This class was a helpful overview of the manikin and how simulation is run and debriefed.
    A. Strongly agree   B. Agree   C. Undecided   D. Disagree   E. Strongly Disagree

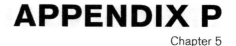

Faculty Simulation Orientation Evaluation *(cont'd)*

12. A helpful suggestion or addition I have that might make the class more beneficial is:_____

_____

_____

_____

_____

_____

_____

_____

13. Something I might omit from the class might be: _____

_____

_____

_____

_____

_____

_____

14. Additional comments: _____

_____

_____

_____

_____

_____

_____

_____

ENGAGING THE LEARNER ACTIVITIES

STUDENT-CENTERED LEARNING ACTIVITIES
LINKED TO PROFESSIONAL AND NCLEX® STANDARDS

Resources Needed for Activities	The Eight-Step Approach for Teaching Clinical Nursing (Zager, Manning & Herman, 2017)	The Eight-Step Approach for Student Clinical Success (Zager, Manning & Herman, 2017)
Standards	**Faculty Instructions**	**Student Instructions**
Management of Care Organize workload to manage time effectively. Serve as a resource person to other staff.	**Scavenger Hunt for Simulation** 1. Have students in groups of 2 or 3 find items on a list that is specific to your simulation lab (i.e., the medication cart, provider orders, equipment, how to call the healthcare provider, where to find lab reports, what information they can get from the medical record versus what they need to assess on the manikin, etc.). a. Have the students conduct a tour and show you where items are located in the simulation lab once they have completed their scavenger hunt.	**Scavenger Hunt for Simulation** 1. Work in groups of 2 or 3 to find where the items on the list are located in your simulation lab. a. When you are done, you and your fellow students will conduct a tour for your faculty to show them where the items are located in your simulation lab.
Safety & Infection Control Ensure proper identification of client when providing care. Apply principles of infection control (i.e., hand hygiene). Assure appropriate and safe use of equipment in performing client care.	**First Assessment of Client and Environment** 2. Role model the process. *Have the students practice in pairs and give each other feedback* prior to the simulation and/or clinical. a. Knock on the door before they enter. b. Greet the client and/or family members when they enter the room. c. Introduce themselves. d. Wash their hands. e. Identify the client by two methods. f. Check healthcare provider orders. g. Check the MAR. h. Assess information provided on simulation monitor and equipment in the room (i.e., Foley, IV pump, drains, ambu bag for peds, etc.). i. Perform a safety check (i.e., bedrails, bed in position, call light, etc.). j. Talk aloud their actions, assessment findings, interventions and the response of the client (manikin).	**First Assessment of Client and Environment** 2. Practice in pairs the series of actions necessary when you enter a client's room in simulation and/or clinical for the first assessment of your client and their environment. Practice the actions prior to the simulation and /or clinical. Remind each other of the actions if necessary. a. Knock on door before entering. b. Greet the client and/or family members when you enter. c. Introduce yourself. d. Wash your hands. e. Identify client by 2 methods. f. Check provider orders. g. Check the MAR. h. Assess information provided on simulation monitor and equipment in the room (i.e., Foley, IV pump, drains, ambu bag for peds, etc.). i. Perform a safety check (i.e., bedrails, bed in position, call light, etc.). j. Talk aloud your actions, assessment findings, interventions and the response of the client (manikin).

Deciding When to Use Low- and High-Stakes Simulation

Kate K. Chappell, MSN, APRN, CPNP-PC / Erin McKinney, MN, RN, RNC-OB

IN THIS CHAPTER YOU WILL LEARN ABOUT:

→ Low- and High-Stakes Simulation: Application and Differences

→ Planning Recommendations for High-Stakes Simulation

→ Options for High-Stakes Simulation Grading

→ Recommendations for Feedback When Evaluating Simulation

This chapter will bring to life the definition stated in Chapter 5: "Simulation education is a bridge between classroom learning and real-life clinical experience" (Simulation for Society in Healthcare, 2016). Simulation provides a safe environment for students to learn, make mistakes, and practice what they have learned. When students make mistakes, they see the results of their interventions and increase the depth of their learning (Simulation for Society in Healthcare 2016). They connect assessments and interventions with outcomes that are necessary for safe and effective care.

Chapter 5 discussed the components of simulation. It is important to know that there are two ways to approach simulation: low-stakes and high-stakes:

✦ **Low-stakes simulation** is ungraded and used primarily for learning experiences and formative evaluation of student progress. Low-stakes builds student comfort with simulation and with clinical skills or situations. It is overall a less stressful student experience. It provides constructive feedback for the student to be able to improve (NLN-SIRC, 2013).

✦ **High-stakes simulation** is used for summative evaluation of student readiness or competence for course-specific skills or content, evaluation of program progress, program objectives/nursing readiness in final clinical course and determining student need for clinical skills remediation. "High-stakes refers to the outcome or consequences of the process" (Meakim, Boese, Decker, Franklin, Gloe, Lioce, Sando, & Borum, 2013).

The two approaches of simulation have distinct purposes. The focus in low-stakes simulation is on reinforcement of learning. The focus on high-stakes simulation is assessment of students' competency. Prior to high-stakes simulation, the student needs to experience the learning aspect of simulation. Recognizing key differences in these two uses of simulation is important when planning to incorporate high-stakes simulation into your program. Deciding to use graded (high-stakes) simulation needs to be a thoughtful, planned process. Graded simulations are called "high stakes" because that is how the students feel! All simulations, either low- or high-stake, need to be based on the curriculum and practice standards.

Tables are used in this chapter to organize the information on the variations in simulation. The tables are:

+ Table 1: Low-Stakes and High-Stakes Simulation: Applications and Differences

+ Table 2: Planning Recommendations for High-Stakes Simulation

+ Table 3: Options for High-Stakes Simulation Grading

+ Table 4: Strategies for Student Feedback in High-Stakes Simulation

Table 1 displays the application, advantages, and limitations of each type of simulation to guide you in your decision making about which one to use.

TABLE 1: LOW-STAKES AND HIGH-STAKES SIMULATION: APPLICATIONS AND DIFFERENCES

Low-Stakes (ungraded) Simulation	Applications	Advantages	Limitations
Low-stakes is primarily used for learning experiences and formative evaluation of student progress.	• Clinical skill practice, either before or after clinical time with clients. • High risk, low occurrences in clinical situations. • Clinical settings/ roles students may not get exposure to (i.e., home health, hospice, or school nursing, etc.).	• Builds student comfort with simulation, clinical skills and/or clinical situations. • Less stressful for the student. • Allows flexibility in setup of simulation (i.e., time for simulation, number of students in scenario, number of faculty available).	• Can be difficult to evaluate students' decision making because some students will take ungraded scenario less seriously, taking clinical actions they never would in real setting. • Students may come less prepared for the simulation.
High-Stakes (graded) Simulation	**Applications**	**Advantages**	**Limitations**
High-stakes is for course specific skills or content, evaluation of program progress, program objectives/nursing readiness in final clinical course, and determining student need for clinical skills remediation.	• Competency evaluation of course-specific skills and/or content. • Determine student need for clinical skills remediation. • Evaluation of student progress, moving from beginning level courses to higher complexity level courses in the program curriculum.	• Course leaders can evaluate students across clinical groups. • Course leaders can see learning strengths and weaknesses across groups. • Course leaders can evaluate students' clinical performance under pressure.	• Student performance may be affected by high level of stress (See Table 2 in this chapter). • Students may share scenario information compromising the simulation and results in unfair grading. • To maintain scenario integrity, it is recommended to have 2 or more simulations of similar complexity and concepts to use on different days. • Each scenario that is run for every participant, must be consistent with the prescribed script to ensure fairness. • Without proper training, multiple facilitators can inadvertently change the perceived priorities of the scenario thus impacting the evaluation of the students' performance. • During a simulation that is focused on a client with COPD presenting with the intended priority of shortness of breath, a faculty member voicing for the client constantly complains of pain thus inadvertently redirects the student's thinking. This example of a faculty dialogue during simulation changes the priority from SOB to pain.

TABLE 2: PLANNING RECOMMENDATIONS FOR HIGH-STAKES SIMULATION

Planning Component	Strategies	Comments/Suggestions
When to Schedule High-Stakes Simulation	• Scheduling should be based on the content and clinical experience the students have had. • High-stakes simulations require that students have more than a one-time exposure to the didactic content and skills that will be graded. • Clear expectations must be communicated.	• Options for hands-on learning of skills and critical thinking may include direct clinical experiences, case studies, or low-stakes simulation and didactic content.

Schedule to Decrease Student Stress	• Avoid having ONLY high-stakes simulations in a course.
	
	• Include at least 1 low-stakes simulation experience prior to the high-stakes.
	
	• Schedule graded simulation/activities during a less busy time in the students' semester.
	
	• Allow students to sign up for their choice of time based on the availability of the lab and faculty schedules.
		• Times to avoid when scheduling high-stakes simulation:
		
		  o The day of or the day before a major test.
		
		  o The end of a full clinical day when students are tired.
		
		  o After a long break, (i.e., spring break, etc.).

Prepare Students for Simulation	• Schedule practice sessions with flexibility to meet the students' needs and decide if the simulation will be optional or required using a different scenario than the graded scenario.
	
	• Components for student practice sessions:
	
	  o Manikin functioning
	  o Room set up
	  o Location of supplies
	  o Format/timing of scenarios
	  o Performance level expectations (i.e., getting report, expected to do focused assessment, etc.)
	  o Equipment that will be used during simulation
	  o Clinical resources student would need, stethoscope, lab or drug books
		• Familiarity with the flow of the simulation process, skills and equipment during practice sessions will improve the assessment of the students' skill and decision making abilities.
		
		• A video of someone going through the steps and time frames of the simulation can also be a helpful preparation tool for students.
		
		• Decisions about the use of cell phones and other resources during the high-stake simulation need to be decided and communicated to the students before the simulation.

Table 1 described how both low- and high-stakes simulation offer opportunities for student learning. Faculty leaders should choose low-stakes or high-stakes based on the goals of the simulation. Careful planning will ensure a positive and successful experience for both student and faculty.

The planning for high-stakes simulation described in Table 2 guides you in your next decision: if the grade will be pass/fail or a numeric/letter grade. Evaluation criteria for both approaches should focus on course objectives, competencies for safe and effective care, and standards of practice (i.e., patient safety and NCLEX® activities). Never plan a simulation for "nice-to-know" information. It should always be standard-based. All grading tools or rubrics should be piloted to promote grading consistency. Evaluation of the tools is an ongoing process to continually fine-tune to the objectives of the scenario.

Table 3 will provide you with options for high-stakes simulation grading and discuss how to develop criteria for both pass/fail and graded scenarios. The following are some additional recommendations for both low-stakes and high-stakes grading that help ensure fair and consistent grading.

+ Minimize the number of faculty grading any one scenario.

+ Conduct a grading reliability exercise (using a recorded scenario) before grading students, particularly important with new graders or a new scenario.

+ Assign experienced faculty to the role of grader when possible.

+ Remain flexible in first run of graded scenario. You may need to adjust points for different actions based on how students perform. They may perform actions you did not initially anticipate in your grading rubric.

+ Wait to release grades until all students have completed the scenario to avoid having to change grades later based on needed adjustments.

+ Record graded simulations when possible in case the course leader needs to review prior to assigning a final grade or to support a grading decision. If it is not possible to record a graded scenario, two faculty graders are highly recommended to assure fairness.

+ If the high-stakes simulation determines whether the student passes the course, the simulation **must** either be recorded or graded by a minimum of two faculty members.

TABLE 3: OPTIONS FOR HIGH-STAKES SIMULATION GRADING

Grading Approach	Strategies	Comments/Suggestions
Pass/Fail Grading Criteria (Refer to Appendix A—Example of a Pass/Fail Grading Checklist for Infant Cardiopulmonary Resuscitation)	Consider for Pass/Fail: • End-of-course evaluations such as Health Assessment where the focus is on a skill. • Competency testing of core skills for a course or across a program (i.e., medication administration, infection control, etc.). • Create a checklist with clearly defined evaluation criteria for each pass/fail item. (Refer to Appendix A—Example of a Pass/Fail Grading Checklist for Infant Cardiopulmonary Resuscitation) • Predetermine the number of critical criteria that are a "must pass" for the scenario. This information is not shared with the students and only faculty graders should be informed. • A student's overall pass/fail grade should be based on objective and not subjective criteria (i.e., "adequate communication" or "therapeutic approach", etc.).	• Each student's required action should be explicitly specified to ensure the objectives are met and grading is fair. • Sharing the "must pass" criteria with students could create over-analysis of how they are doing during the simulation and affect their performance. • Students often assume points are being deducted for everything and become more anxious than if they just focus on giving safe, competent care. • Items related to subjective concepts need a specific benchmark (i.e., instead of "adequate communication with team members and client," use "minimum of 3 SBAR components used to call the provider," etc.).
Numerical Grading Rubric *Designed for 1 simulation or station using base points.* (Refer to Appendix B—Grading Rubric Using Base Points)	Consider Numerical Grading Rubric for: • Evaluating complex or multi-step decision making processes. • End-of-course evaluations for advanced or specialty courses. (Refer to Appendix C—Example of Multi-client Simulation with Multiple Diagnoses and Concepts for the End of Course or Capstone Experience) • Prepare a grading rubric ahead of time to guide the faculty graders. (Refer to Appendix B—Grading Rubric Using Base Points) • The grading rubric points that determine the numeric grade should be standardized objective criteria and not subjective.	• Anticipate students may take different actions or paths that are not the objective of the scenario. o Assign points for components done/not done as clear and specific as possible. (i.e., in a CPR scenario, add or deduct points for each step of CPR, the technique used during CPR and recognition of when it is time to stop CPR).

TABLE 3: OPTIONS FOR HIGH-STAKES SIMULATION GRADING *(cont'd)*

Grading Approach	Strategies	Comments/Suggestions
Numeric Grading Rubric *Designed for multi-station simulations.*	• Prepare a grading rubric ahead of time to guide the faculty graders. (Refer to Appendix D–Grading Rubric for Multi-Station Simulation) o Appendix C (Example of a Multi-Client Simulation with Multiple Diagnoses and Concepts for the End of Course or Capstone Experience) includes grading of high-stakes simulation with the pediatric response scenario, pediatric growth assessment skill station and the medication administration skill station. • The grading rubric points that determine the numeric grade should be standardized objective criteria and not subjective. • Include in the criteria for graded points, any skill stations (i.e., medication stations or other non-live scenario components, etc.).	• Students may be less anxious if grade is not dependent on one 10-minute graded scenario. • Graded skill stations provide an opportunity to test additional skills in timed and untimed activities. (Refer to Appendix E–Pediatric Growth Assessment Skill Station with Grading Rubric) and (Appendix F–Medication Administration Skill Station with Grading Rubric)

Table 4 provides guidance and strategies for giving effective feedback with high-stakes that will minimize frustration and facilitate students to learn from the experience. Often in high-stakes, the formal debrief format may not be used; instead students are given feedback about their performance and their grade. The table also provides guidance for when a student's performance was unsuccessful.

TABLE 4: STRATEGIES FOR STUDENT FEEDBACK IN HIGH-STAKES SIMULATION

	Strategies	Comments/Suggestions
Content of Feedback	• Focus on areas of strength and areas needing improvement. • Avoid disclosing all details of grading and of the scenario to retain the integrity of the scenario.	• Reviewing detailed listing of points deducted is not feasible for multiple students or groups. • Posting or sending grading rubrics to students compromises the scenario's use in future semesters.
Timing of Feedback	• Provide feedback after the students finish their simulation. *Options:* • Immediate general feedback following the simulation to the individual or small group on areas of strength and those that need improvement. • Combined debrief session with several groups. (Refer to Chapter 5, Table 1– Planning Simulation) • Feedback can also be provided to the class via a short video or other means to guide students' self-reflection.	• Immediate feedback promotes learning and reduces anxiety for those who have completed the simulation and for the students that are waiting simulation. • If an individual makes a critical error in a small group scenario, provide the feedback to the individual prior to the group debrief to maintain privacy. • More specific detail can be provided after all students have finished their simulation and grades are posted. However, it is still important to maintain the integrity of the scenario and grading rubric.
Timing of Pass/ Non-Passing Notifications	• Provide performance status (pass or fail) as soon as possible.	• All students should be notified of their grade in the same time frame. • Frequently this information may not be available immediately due to multiple days of simulation for large groups or the need for a course leader to review any non-passing attempts. • State when and how an initial "pass/fail" notification will be provided (i.e., via email within 48 hours) followed by posting of finalized grades. • If there will be a delay in the notification, that should be included in the prep information.

TABLE 4: STRATEGIES FOR STUDENT FEEDBACK
IN HIGH-STAKES SIMULATION *(cont'd)*

	Strategies	Comments/Suggestions
Consequences for Non-Passing Attempts	• Consequences of a non-passing simulation grade, should be clearly stated in the course syllabi. • Consider allowing a second opportunity to pass the evaluation. The second opportunity with guidelines should be clearly noted in syllabus.	• Avoid misunderstandings of how a non-passing score will affect their final clinical grade or their course success. Be upfront! • Simulation can be stressful. With an ultimate goal of student learning and competence, a second opportunity allows students a path to success.
Repeats for non-passing attempts	• Specifically describe the grading procedure for re-attempts in the course syllabi. *Grading options for a second attempt* • Average the initial and second attempt grades. OR • Set a maximum grade that any successful second attempt could earn.	
Strengthening/ Remediation Opportunity	• Offer a remediation session to further strengthen skills, using the same or a different scenario. • The remediation may be required for all students who needed a second attempt and an optional for other students who desire to strengthen their skills.	• Remediation is especially recommended when the students will have additional high-stakes simulation in future courses.

In order for students to learn, they must receive feedback for every simulation experience, whether low- or high-stakes. Without feedback, students may think they correctly managed a situation when, in fact, their actions were unsafe or incomplete. Feedback also allows students to recognize areas for improvement and know where they are competent.

For high-stakes simulation, faculty should be cautious with specific feedback to avoid compromising scenario information and critical points on the grading rubric. It is important to handle a student's potential disappointment in their grade or their non-passing of the evaluation respectfully. Students become frustrated when they do not receive feedback and may feel the grading was unfair.

We recommend, based on our experience, that the feedback method instead of the formal debrief be used when the scenario is graded. As stated earlier, the student's anxiety is high with graded simulation. Appropriate feedback makes all the difference for the student so that learning takes place.

CONCLUSION

The decision about high- or low-stakes simulation should be based on the objectives of the scenario and the course outcomes. The tables in this chapter have described the advantages of each. The most valuable part of simulation for students is the feedback they receive from you. Learning will not take place without it. Simulation with appropriate feedback assists students to gain the clinical-reasoning skills necessary for them to become safe, practicing nurses.

Example of a Pass/Fail Grading Checklist for
Infant Cardiopulmonary Resuscitation

Student: _____ Evaluator: _____ Date: _____

This checklist assesses competency around one skill: **in-hospital infant CPR.** (Refer to Appendix D in Chapter 5: Example of an Original Scenario Packet Pediatric Emergency Response.) Stop the scenario at five minutes *or* when all of the skills below have been satisfactorily completed–whichever happens first.

Competency	Circle the assessment for each competency. 00 = automatic fail items. *If any of these essentials are not done, regardless of total points, assessment of competency is non-passing.*** **0** = not done **1** = done
Handwashing or hand sanitizer upon entering room	0 1
Assesses responsiveness	0 1
Calls Code Blue Jr./Emergency Response within 2 minutes	0 1
Assesses airway and breathing	0 1
Positions airway *(head tilt/chin lift without excessive tilting of infant's head)*	0 1
Starts rescue breathing via Ambu-bag in 1st minute of scenario**	00 1
Ambu-bag is attached to oxygen 10 Liters/minute or higher	0 1
Assesses pulse at brachial site for infant *(okay if uses other sites or auscultates to confirm low/absent HR)*	0 1
Starts chest compressions within 2 minutes of scenario**	00 1
Chest compressions with two-finger, thumbs encircled, or one-handed method	0 1
Chest compressions register as adequate on manikin monitor *(or appear to be 1/3 the depth of manikin's chest)***	00 1
Compression to breaths in ratio of 15:2 (2-rescuer) or 30:2 (1-rescuer)	0 1
Compression rate at least 100 /minute**	00 1
Continues compressions until client heart rate at least 90/minute	0 1
Continues rescue breaths while client not breathing/low RR for age** *(if stop scenario before other treatment, this infant will not breathe during scenario; rescue breaths should continue through scenario)*	00 1
Comments:	**TOTAL No. of 00:** _____ *(automatic non-passing if one or more 00)* **TOTAL No. of 0:** _____ *(predetermined number of 0's for non-passing: ___)*

APPENDIX B

Grading Rubric Using Base Points

For use in high-stakes simulation experience of The Pediatric Respiratory Failure Scenario
(Chapter 5, Appendix D: Example of an Original Scenario Packet
Pediatric Emergency Response)

ALL scores at bottom include the BASELINE 70 points. Circle the applicable points.

Safety/Infection Preparation *(circle all that apply)*	Emergency Equipment Check (ambu-bag, mask, suction, O_2 suction)	+0.5
	Verifies IV site and IVFs	+0.5
	Handwashing/Foam	+0.5
	ID check	+0.5
Pre-Scenario History Gathering *(circle all that apply)*	Asks Reporting Nurse at least two pertinent questions to situation	+1
	Asks mother at least two pertinent questions to situation	+1
CPR Initiation *only points if no prompt during provider contact* *(only circle ONE)*	Starts compressions & ambu-bag within 1 minute	+4
	Starts compressions & ambu-bag within 2 minutes	+3
	Starts compression & rescue breaths within 2 minutes OR ONLY compression or rescue breaths OR CPR started after 2-minute point	+2
	Prompt required to start CPR	+0
Calling for Help *(only circle ONE)*	Calls Code Blue Jr. within 30 seconds without prompting	+3
	Calls Code Blue Jr. within 2 minutes without prompting OR changes to Code Blue from Rapid Response without prompting	+2
	Calls Rapid Response within 2 minutes without prompting OR calls Code sometime after 2 minutes	+1
	Code called after prompt by provider or no Code called	+0
Assessments/Interventions *(circle all that apply)*	Assessed or repositioned airway OR Questioned airway patency	+1
	Suctioned client	+1
	Repositioned for re-shunt attempt	+1
	Temperature obtained without prompt	+1
	Blood glucose obtained without prompt	+1
CPR Technique	CPR technique by student correct per observation and/or Simulator	+1
	Student CPR technique incorrect	+0
CPR Continuity *(only circle ONE)*	No unneeded CPR stops and effective coordination	+2
	1 stop or some ineffective periods	+0.5
	Multiple stops or ineffective periods	+0

Grading Rubric Using Base Points *(cont'd)*

ABC Reassessment	Reassesses ABC's at least once during scenario	+2
	No ABC reassessment	+0
Delegation	Delegating full CPR responsibility to one nurse (if 2 total in room) or to two nurses (if 3 total in room)	+1
	Not delegated to one; all in room focusing only on CPR for entire scenario	+0
Provider Contact	Calls provider prior to 4 minutes	+1
	Calls provider after 4 minutes	+0.5
	Provider not called ("Delayed" Code team will call at 4 minutes to prompt)	+0
SBAR *(only circle ONE)*	Correct SBAR on provider call	+2
	Missing 1 component of SBAR or inaccuracies	+1
	SBAR not used, multiple missing components	+0
Temperature Management *(only circle ONE; circle nothing if temperature not addressed)*	Places infant under Radiant Heat Warmer with eye covers, diaper, and no blanket/clothes	+4
	Places infant under Radiant Heat Warmer without eye covers and/or with blanket/clothes	+3
	Bundles infant in (stated) warmed blankets with socks and hat	+3
	Bundles infant in (stated) warmed blankets without clothing added	+1
Teamwork	Strong collaboration and teamwork throughout	Give 0 to +3
	Lapses in teamwork, decreased collaboration	
Unsafe Action	Possibly dangerous action taken during care (oral glucose, etc.) For each:	-2
Unordered Medications *(circle all that apply)*	Changes ordered meds or IVFs without orders	-2
	Administers epinephrine or atropine at safe dose without an order	-3
	Administers epinephrine or atropine at unsafe/unverified dose without an order	-4
	Administers any other medication without an order	-6

Baseline: 70

Total Pts From Above: _____

Final Group Score: _____

May give up to +2 points if a student provided exceptional leadership or added clinical expertise beyond expectations or subtract up to -10 points if a student did not fully participate/contribute or was a significant teamwork barrier.

<u>Final Individual Scores:</u>

Student: _____   Score: _____

Student: _____   Score: _____

Student: _____   Score: _____

APPENDIX C

EXAMPLE OF A MULTI-CLIENT SIMULATION WITH MULTIPLE DIAGNOSES AND CONCEPTS FOR THE END OF COURSE OR CAPSTONE EXPERIENCE

Assessment of Clinical Reasoning, Competency and Prioritization

The multi-client simulation is an exceptional way to evaluate a student's mastery of content and their ability to prioritize care. This can be done at the end of each course and/or as a senior capstone simulation that includes content across the curriculum.

The learning outcomes of multi-client scenarios include *prioritization* of which client should be seen first based on the clinical findings given in the client's report. It also includes initiation of priority assessments and interventions based on standards that are appropriate for the care required. A representative group of clients with a variety of medical diagnoses that include multiple priority concepts can be set up as simulation scenarios in the simulation lab in separate rooms. Selection of clients should include diagnoses that are associated with high risk for potential complications commonly seen in the clinical area (i.e., deep vein thrombosis, post-partum bleeding, hypoglycemic episode, and fluid and electrolyte imbalances, etc.). This selection of clients helps students to reinforce safe-care competencies and assists the instructor to identify the challenges.

Students can be assigned individually or in pairs for this simulation. The components of the multi-client simulation exercise include a start-of-shift report on three to five clients. The students, after hearing report, select the priority client they wish to see first and provide direct client care until the simulation is complete. This process allows the clinical instructor to evaluate students' ability to process large amounts of client data and use clinical decision-making to identify the priority client based on the system-specific assessment findings of each client.

The guidelines for simulation are followed as outlined in the tables in Chapter 5. Ideally students would see all of the clients included in the report. If that is not possible due to resources, the students are directed to the correct client if they do not choose the priority client.

The grading rubric for low- or high-stakes simulation begins with a baseline grade and credit is added for each correct assessment and/or interventions. Points are not subtracted unless the students perform unsafe behaviors or are negligent in their care. The simulation exercise includes four main sections:

- Selection of the correct priority client based on the initial report received.

- Completion of specific assessments related to the client's changing status following patient safety and practice standards.

- Completion of specific interventions related to the client's changing status following patient safety and practice standards.

- Communication with the client and a SBAR format communication either to the healthcare provider by phone or to the handoff nurse at the completion of the scenario.

GRADING RUBRIC FOR MULTI-STATION SIMULATION

For use in high-stakes simulation experience in one scheduled session, including:

1. The Pediatric Respiratory Failure Scenario in Chapter 5, Appendix D *(maximum pts: 80)*
2. Medication Administration Skill Station in Chapter 6, Appendix F *(maximum pts: 14)*
3. Pediatric Growth Assessment Skill Station in Chapter 6, Appendix E *(maximum pts: 10)*

Points earned across all experiences will add to one total score *(maximum potential: 104)*

1. Circle the applicable points for the Pediatric Respiratory Failure Scenario:

Safety/Infection Preparation *(circle all that apply)*	Emergency Equipment Check (ambu-bag, mask, suction, O_2 suction)	+2
	Verifies IV site and IVFs	+2
	Handwashing/Foam	+2
	ID check	+2
Pre-Scenario History Gathering *(circle all that apply)*	Asks Reporting Nurse at least two pertinent questions to situation	+2
	Asks mother at least two pertinent questions to situation	+2
CPR Initiation *only points if no prompt during provider contact* *(only circle ONE)*	Starts compressions & ambu-bag within 1 minute	+8
	Starts compressions & ambu-bag within 2 minutes	+6
	Starts compression & rescue breaths within 2 minutes OR ONLY compression or rescue breaths OR CPR started after 2-minute point	+4
	Prompt required to start CPR	+0
Calling for Help *(only circle ONE)*	Calls Code Blue Jr. within 30 seconds without prompting	+8
	Calls Code Blue Jr. within 2 minutes without prompting OR changes to Code Blue from Rapid Response without prompting	+6
	Calls Rapid Response within 2 minutes without prompting OR calls Code sometime after 2 minutes	+4
	Code called after prompt by provider or no Code called	+0
Assessments/Interventions *(circle all that apply)*	Assessed or repositioned airway OR Questioned airway patency	+3
	Suctioned client	+2
	Repositioned for re-shunt attempt	+2
	Temperature obtained without prompt	+3
	Blood glucose obtained without prompt	+3
CPR Technique	CPR technique by student correct per observation and/or Simulator	+5
	Student CPR technique incorrect	+0
CPR Continuity *(only circle ONE)*	No unneeded CPR stops and effective coordination	+5
	1 stop or some ineffective periods	+3
	Multiple stops or ineffective periods	+0

cont'd on next page

GRADING RUBRIC FOR MULTI-STATION SIMULATION *(cont'd)*

ABC Reassessment	Reassesses ABC's at least once during scenario	+6
	No ABC reassessment	+0
Delegation	Delegating full CPR responsibility to one nurse (if 2 total in room) or to two nurses (if 3 total in room)	+2
	Not delegated to one; all in room focusing only on CPR for entire scenario	+0
Provider Contact	Calls provider prior to 4 minutes	+2
	Calls provider after 4 minutes	+1
	Provider not called ("Delayed" Code team will call at 4 minutes to prompt)	+0
SBAR *(only circle ONE)*	Correct SBAR on provider call	+4
	Missing 1 component of SBAR or inaccuracies	+2
	SBAR not used, multiple missing components	+0
Temperature Management *(only circle ONE; circle nothing if temperature not addressed)*	Places infant under Radiant Heat Warmer with eye covers, diaper, and no blanket/clothes	+10
	Places infant under Radiant Heat Warmer without eye covers and/or with blanket/clothes	+7
	Bundles infant in (stated) warmed blankets with socks and hat	+7
	Bundles infant in (stated) warmed blankets without clothing added	+5
Teamwork	Strong collaboration and teamwork throughout	Give 0 to +5
	Lapses in teamwork, decreased collaboration	
Unsafe Action	Possibly dangerous action taken during care (oral glucose, etc.) **For each:**	-4
Unordered Medications *(circle all that apply)*	Changes ordered meds or IVFs without orders	-4
	Administers epinephrine or atropine at safe dose without an order	-5
	Administers epinephrine or atropine at unsafe/unverified dose without an order	-6
	Administers any other medication without an order	-8

Total Points From Above (Final Group Score): _____

May give up to +2 points if a student provided exceptional leadership or added clinical expertise beyond expectations or subtract up to -10 points if a student did not fully participate/contribute or was a significant teamwork barrier.

<u>Final Individual Scores for Scenario:</u>

Student: _____ Score: _____

Student: _____ Score: _____

Student: _____ Score: _____

GRADING RUBRIC FOR MULTI-STATION SIMULATION *(cont'd)*

Final Scores from Multi-station Simulation Experience

Student: _____

1. Scenario Score from above: _____

2. Medication Administration Skill Station Points (using rubric in Ch. 6, Appendix F): _____

3. Pediatric Growth Assessment Skill Station Points (using rubric in Ch. 6, Appendix E): _____

Total Final Student Score: _____

Student: _____

1. Scenario Score from above: _____

2. Medication Administration Skill Station Points (using rubric in Ch. 6, Appendix F): _____

3. Pediatric Growth Assessment Skill Station Points (using rubric in Ch. 6, Appendix E): _____

Total Final Student Score: _____

Student: _____

1. Scenario Score from above: _____

2. Medication Administration Skill Station Points (using rubric in Ch. 6, Appendix F): _____

3. Pediatric Growth Assessment Skill Station Points (using rubric in Ch. 6, Appendix E): _____

Total Final Student Score: _____

APPENDIX E

PEDIATRIC GROWTH ASSESSMENT SKILL STATION WITH RUBRIC

Instructor Directions and Answer Key

Provide a copy of *Client Information and Questions* (the next page of the appendix) and a copy of the correct growth chart for each student or student pair. (See below for references for growth charts.) You can laminate these for repeated use with multiple groups.

- The Center for Disease Control (CDC) website offers online modules that are useful for this skill station or for pre-clinical independent work. Modules cover the use of CDC growth charts, measurement in special populations, and common measurement errors. (Refer to http://www.cdc.gov/nccdphp/dnpao/growthcharts/)

- Another resource for practice on the growth charts is the World Health Organization (WHO) and CDC Growth Charts. (Refer to https://cdc.gov/growthcharts/index.htm)

To use this skill station as part of a low-stakes clinical experience, first address these points for accurate growth charting:

- Demonstrate charting growth by drawing a line from exact age crossed with line from measurement number.

- Discuss answer documentation. Examples: If a plot point is right in a line, document as "10th percentile," for instance. If a plot point is between two lines, state as "between 10th and 25th," for instance. If a plot point is above or below charted areas, document as "above 95th percentile," for instance.
  - Estimating between percentiles or rounding to the nearest percentile is inconsistent with CDC guidance.

- Growth charting is about patterns. If a child's percentiles move by more than 2 lines across different dates, this pattern suggests growth delay, abnormal acceleration or excess weight gain.

- When assessing BMI-for-age, a child is considered overweight when at the 90th or higher BMI percentile-for-age. This is a more accurate measure than BMI for kids.

To use this skill station as part of a high-stakes multi-station simulation:

Students need prior content, such as the CDC modules, and prior hands-on work, such as a low-stakes skill station or practice items. Set a time limit *(suggestion: 15 minutes)*. Students turn in answers on separate paper for later grading. The grading rubric for this skill station is the last page of this appendix. Also, Appendix D (Grading Rubric for Multi-Station Simulation) is a combined rubric that can be used with this skill station, a medication station, and a simulation scenario.

Answer Key:

1. What is the height-percentile-for-age today?
   Answer: between 25-50th percentiles

2. What is the weight-percentile-for-age today?
   Answer: between 90-95th percentiles

3. What is the body-mass-index-for-age percentile today?
   Answer: > 95th percentile

4. What would be your specific suggestions in the plan of care? What information would you share with the provider?
   Answer: List specific actions for healthy changes (activities such as evening walks, playing active games, yard work, and diet changes as a family or cooking healthy meals together).

5. What information would you share with the provider?
   Answer: Notify provider child's BMI-for-age indicates obesity.

PEDIATRIC GROWTH ASSESSMENT SKILL STATION WITH RUBRIC *(cont'd)*

Skill Station: Pediatric Growth Assessment (Client Information and Questions)

Use current growth chart for 2-20-year-old females at *www.cdc.gov* for answering questions.

Client: S.K., 4½-year-old female. No history of chronic illnesses.

Time setting of appointment: April

Today's measurements: Height: 102 cm   Weight: 21 kg

At last visit (4 years old): Height: 102 cm   Weight: 19 kg

3-year-old visit: Height: 93 cm   Weight: 15.5 kg

2-year-old visit (first visit at this location. No earlier records available): Height: 84 cm Weight: 12 kg

Address the following questions:

1. What is the height-percentile-for-age today?

2. What is the weight-percentile-for-age today?

3. What is the body-mass-index-for-age percentile today?

4. What would be your specific suggestions in the plan of care?

5. What information would you share with the provider?

cont'd on next page

APPENDIX E
Chapter 6

PEDIATRIC GROWTH ASSESSMENT SKILL STATION WITH RUBRIC *(cont'd)*

Student: _____ Evaluator: _____ Date: _____

Once student turns in work, student cannot return to work space. Take student answer sheet and ALL notes from student when complete and staple to this sheet. Do not discuss correctness of answers with the student.

Question and Responses	Points (no partial points beyond what is listed). **Clearly circle and choose the one best option for each item.**
Height percentile-for-age: 25–50th percentile 25th percentile 50th percentile A number between 25th and 50th (i.e., 30th) All other answers	+2 +1 +1 +1 0
Weight percentile-for-age: 90–95th percentile 95th percentile 90th percentile Above 95th percentile A number between 90th and 95th (i.e., 92nd) All other answers	+2 +1 +1 +1 +1 0
BMI percentile-for-age: Above 95th percentile 95th percentile 90–95th percentile A number above 95th (i.e., 98th) All other answers	+2 +1 +.5 +.5 0
Next step in plan of care. **Healthy lifestyle actions:** 3+ actions, at least 1 with family involvement 2 actions, at least 1 with family involvement 1 action with family involvement **Healthy lifestyle actions:** 3+ actions focused on the child 2 actions focused on the child 1 action focused on the child General answer on weight loss, diet, or exercise No concerns for BMI, concerns for weight being too low, or other incorrect interpretation	 +2.5 +2 +1.5 +1.5 +1 +.5 +1 0
Provider Communication: Plans to notify provider child is obese Plans to notify provider child is overweight Plans to notify, no specifics on meaning of BMI Answer does not include notifying provider Answer includes weight/BMI being normal or low	+1.5 +1 +.5 0 0

Comments: TOTAL PTS: _____/MAX PTS: 10

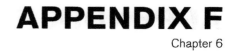

MEDICATION ADMINISTRATION SKILL STATION

Table of Contents

cont'd on next page

MEDICATION ADMINISTRATION SKILL STATION *(cont'd)*

Evaluator Overview and Instructions

Evaluators: read completely PRIOR to beginning the scenario!

At this station, students will each sit at an individual table and review the client scenario. They will then prepare the medications due at this time and also recognize any orders needed/due that need questioning/ verifying. As students soon to be licensed and practicing, these are important skills for them to be able to perform independently.

This station is most successful if planned for a larger space with several individual work spaces. You will need a proctor to monitor; a common cart or table containing medication supplies; and an adjoining room where the instructor evaluator can receive answers and information from each individual student. This is one version of a scenario for the station; additional versions with similar difficulty and similar details can be created to allow for variation across multiple clinical days to preserve scenario and grading integrity, especially when using as part of a high-stakes simulation.

Because this scenario may be used on multiple days with other students, *do not discuss or indicate with facial expressions whether their answers are correct, incorrect, etc.* If a student asks how they did, tell them the course coordinators will share a summary related to this station with the class when check offs are complete. The coordinators will have score sheets for review if needed later.

Process for Medication Administration Station Evaluators:

Up to 4 students will come into middle room to start this station at a time; the proctor in the room will help ensure *the students stay separate in their work space and do not have any materials of any kind with them.*

At each individual work space:

- Laminated copy of the 3-page student scenario
- Note paper
- Medication guide and lab test guide books

The time limit for preparation is 20 minutes (prior to coming to evaluator to report and show their prepared medications). Between you and the proctor, monitor time and, at 15 minutes, go to individual to inform them they must check off in 5 minutes. If student has not finished prep by 20 minutes, they are to come to you and present what they have and will receive credit accordingly. Please note on grading rubric at bottom if a student went to 20 minute time limit. *For fairness across grading multiple students, no student can be allowed to go beyond the time limit.*

If you wish to use this skill station in conjunction with other pediatric activities for a high-stakes simulation evaluation (Refer to Appendix D—Grading Rubric for Multi-Station Simulation) for a combined rubric with this skill station, a pediatric growth assessment skill station, and a simulation scenario.

MEDICATION ADMINISTRATION SKILL STATION *(cont'd)*

Evaluator Overview and Instructions *(cont'd)*

When checking off, students may have notes from their prep work and should have the scenario sheets and any medications they plan on giving to their client at this time.

Step 1: Student begins to discuss medication administration. For ALL, regardless of real time, **it is 8:30 AM**. The evaluation sheets are designed with the "correct" medication to administer at the top. If students first talk about items they are questioning, do not interrupt their flow; the grading is farther toward bottom of sheet. When/if they are presenting the "correct" medication, you can see in the top rows the areas they should definitely discuss. If they don't spontaneously provide all areas, **use only the questions on the evaluation sheet to prompt student to demonstrate knowledge** to determine credit for areas of right drug, dose, route, etc. on the sheet. Using the same questions helps maintain consistent and fair grading not based on different evaluators' questions.

Circle their points for each row as you go—don't try to remember after each student leaves!

Use only the point values provided as options on the sheet; guidance on appropriate scoring is in the information on left side. Follow consistently for overall fairness across check off days. If there is a student response that you feel is a "gray area" not answered by the guidance on the sheet, choose the best option and elaborate under comments. Place any you are unsure of to the side so that course coordinators can determine if any adjustment is warranted.

Step 2: Take students' prep papers from them when they are done reporting to you. The prep papers may NOT leave the station area. Students leaving with notes will result in all points earned in this station being void.

- Staple their notes to back of evaluation sheet.
- Total the points at the bottom. Add a comment if you feel something unusual or noteworthy occurred.
- Return the scenario sheets to any empty prep station for next available student.

Thanks for your help with this station!!

cont'd on next page

MEDICATION ADMINISTRATION SKILL STATION *(cont'd)*

Equipment/Supply Sheet

Use this list to prepare for the skill station.

For the Medication Preparation Table/Cart:

- Bottle of Escitalopram 20 mg tablets (adequate number for students working at station to each give 1 tablet)

- Bottle of Fexofenadine 90 mg tablets (adequate number for students working at station to each give 2 tablets)
  - o You can choose to label as 180 mg tablets but using 90 mg tablets provides evaluation of safe medication administration due to needing more than one tablet to fill order.

- Bottle of Acetaminophen 500 mg tablets (no student should seek to give this, serves as a distractor)

- Medication cups (adequate number for students working at station to each use one)

For the Individual Student Work Spaces in Prep Area:

- Laminated set of Student Scenario Packet

- Medication guide book

- Lab test guide book

- Blank notepaper

For the Faculty Evaluator Space Near Student Prep Area:

- Adequate copies of grading rubric

- Stapler to attach the collected student note pages to grading rubric. (Student note pages should not leave the testing area.)

MEDICATION ADMINISTRATION SKILL STATION *(cont'd)*

Student Instructions to Post in Waiting Area

Read Before Going to Your Work Space!

- You are not allowed to bring any note papers, calculators, or reference materials while at this station and should not leave with any note papers or other materials. Your score may be voided if you leave with note papers or other items.

- Go to an individual work space and review the scenario. Next, prepare your medication administration information and prepare any syringes, pills, etc. you need to give your medications.

- You may use the resources and note paper at your work space. You may use your prep notes while you report to an evaluator.

- You have 20 minutes maximum to prepare to report to an evaluator. The proctor or evaluator will prompt you when you have 5 minutes left.

- At the end of 20 minutes (or earlier if ready), report to an evaluator. Even if you are not completely ready, provide as much of the medication administration as possible. You will not be allowed to take longer than 20 minutes to prepare and will lose points or be unable to complete the station for delaying past the time limit.

- When ready to check off, take the prepared medications, laminated student sheets, and any notes you have made with you to evaluator.

- Evaluator will not indicate whether you are correct with your information to maintain fairness to all students checking off on various days. But, the evaluator may ask you additional scripted questions to provide an opportunity to show what you know for items in the scoring.

- When done, give the evaluator the laminated student sheets and your notes from the station before leaving. Taking any materials or information with you from the station will result in voiding your points from this station.

Provide safe care and follow your medication preparation principles.

You can do this!

cont'd on next page

APPENDIX F

MEDICATION ADMINISTRATION SKILL STATION *(cont'd)*

Student Scenario Packet: Instructions

Student Instructions: You have 20 minutes to review the client information, then prepare medications.

The client has medications due NOW (0830 on medicine administration record). Prepare your medications as if you are taking them to the client's room to give them. Consider your client's current condition in your care.

- Prepare and take all appropriate medications with you to the instructor station when you are ready to administer.

- If there is a medication that you are unable to prepare based on available options, unsafe dose, or other concern, discuss with the instructor as part of your medication administration discussion. You will need to talk them through your medication administration decision-making and procedure on each medication that is due (discuss the 5 rights, how long to infuse if IV, and have it fully prepared, i.e., drawn up in appropriate syringe, diluted if needed, etc.). Discuss concerns such as assessments you need before administering the medications, any calls that are needed to provider, etc., while at the instructor station. No credit will be given for information that is not presented while at the instructor station.

This is an individual station with no collaboration between students. Use clinical resources as allowed by the instructor at the station.

MEDICATION ADMINISTRATION SKILL STATION *(cont'd)*

Student Scenario Packet: Scenario

THE SCENARIO: It is 0800 in an inpatient adolescent psychiatric unit.

Client: Jasmine Allen, 14-year-old African American Female

Weight: 100 lbs.   **Allergy:** NKDA

History: Admitted 4 days ago after 2-day medical stay. 2nd attempted overdose with acetaminophen. Treated with acetylcysteine. No past psychiatric medications. A new medication order received yesterday, to start today, is on MAR.

Diagnoses: Mood Disorder, Seasonal Allergies (takes Allegra at home daily)

Most recent labs *(obtained 5 days ago)*:

CBC: RBC 5 million cells/µL

WBC 9,400 cells/µL

Platelets 266,000 cells/µL

Hemoglobin 11.9 grams/dL

Hematocrit 37%

BMP: Sodium 137 mEq/L   Potassium 3.7 mEq/L

Chloride 97 mEq/L CO_2 21 mEq/L

Glucose 89 mg/dL   Blood Urea Nitrogen 13 mg/dL

Calcium 9.1 mg/dL   Serum Creatinine 0.7 mg/dL

Acetaminophen level: 49 mcg/mL

Today's Assessment (0800): Appears irritable, oriented x 3. Reports eating "only mashed potatoes" last night; refusing breakfast now. Asked how she feels today, states: "No one understands me. Nothing will ever get better." Night shift report: Client repeatedly stated, "I just want everything to stop. Easier to not be here anymore" and "Pills haven't worked. If I try again, I'll try something else."

cont'd on next page

MEDICATION ADMINISTRATION SKILL STATION *(cont'd)*

Student Scenario Packet: Medication Administration Record

Allen, Jasmine   DOB: 2/20/XX   Alleriges: NKDA

	0700–1459	1500–2259	1500–2259
Escitalopram 20 mg PO daily	0830 ____		
Fexofenadine 180 mg PO daily	0830 ____		

MEDICATION ADMINISTRATION SKILL STATION *(cont'd)*

Grading Rubric for Medication Administration Skill Sheet

Student: _____ Evaluator: _____ Date: _____

Once student presents to evaluator, student is not allowed to return to work space. Student is allowed to use notes from prep area. Take ALL notes from student when complete and staple to this sheet.

Do not discuss correctness of choices, etc. with the student. If asked, explain that a summary will be sent to the class after all have completed the activity.

Competency	Points (no partial points beyond what is listed). Circle one choice for each item.			
Presents fexofenadine tablets to give at this **time**. *If student questions fexofenadine order, continue to assess all rights as below. No points for this line item.*	+2		0	
Fexofenadine dose is accurately prepared: **Two 90 mg tablets are given.** *If tablets are 90 mg as on the supply sheet and only 1 is prepared, 0 pts.*	+2		0	
Verbalizes **key considerations prior to administering** and verifies appropriateness in situation. *If not independently stated, ask: "Are there any history or assessments needed prior to giving medication?"* **Key considerations for full credit:** a. Noting client's drug allergy status or if specific past allergy to this medication. b. Verbalizing concern over what the usual dose is that the client takes at home. *Partial credit (+1) if if states only a or b and not both.*	+2	+1	0	
Verbalizes **right drug/right client.** *If not independently stated, ask: "Why is client receiving the medication?"* **Key right Drug response:** seasonal allergies *or* allergies. Verbalizes **evaluation of effect.** *If not independently stated, ask: "What will be the desired effect?"*	+1		0	
Key effect/Expected Outcome: less seasonal allergy response (less coughing, sneezing, runny nose). *If mentions only "less allergic response," ask: "What kinds of responses?"* *If response is still general, 0 pts.*	+1		0	
Verbalizes **right dose.** *If not independently stated, ask: "Is the dose appropriate?"* **Key dose response:** "It is within safe range" *or* "Yes" *or* "It is the highest end of safe." *If states, "I don't know," "not sure," or "too low", 0 pts.*	+2		0	
Verbalizes **right route.** *If not independently stated, evaluator should ask non-leading "What route will be used?"* **Key Route response:** "It is given orally *or* by mouth."	+1		0	
Verbalizes **escitalopram order needs to be questioned** before administration and give the reason. *If student only presents fexofenadine, ask: "Are any other medications on MAR needed at this time or need verifying with provider first?"* **Reasons to question order:** active suicidality with a Black Box warning for teenagers and dose not at the recommended starting level (10 mg). *If only 1 or 2 reasons given, ask: "Any other reasons to question order?"* *If has Escitalopram prepared, allow 7 rights discussion if student begins but do not push for additional information or ask questions.*	+3 (questions order w/2 reasons) +2 (questions order w/1 reason) +1 (questions, no/wrong reason) 0 (not planning on giving or questioning) -3 (planning on giving)			

Comments:

TOTAL PTS: _____/MAX PTS: 14

ENGAGING THE LEARNER ACTIVITIES

Chapter 6

STUDENT-CENTERED LEARNING ACTIVITIES
LINKED TO PROFESSIONAL AND NCLEX® STANDARDS

Resources Needed for Activities	The Eight-Step Approach for Teaching Clinical Nursing (Zager, Manning & Herman, 2017)	The Eight-Step Approach for Student Clinical Success (Zager, Manning & Herman, 2017)
Standards	**Faculty Instructions**	**Student Instructions**

Management of Care
 	
Organize workload to manage time effectively.
	Simulation Preparation Tool
	(Refer to end of Chapter 6, *The Eight-Step Approach for Student Clinical Success*)
	
	1. Have the student complete the Simulation Preparation Tool prior to simulation.
	
	   a. In the debrief, have the students identify information they needed that was missing on their Simulation Preparation Tool.
		Simulation Preparation Tool
		(Refer to end of Chapter 6)
		
		1. Complete the Simulation Preparation Tool on the assigned client scenario prior to simulation.
		
		   a. During debrief, identify any information you needed that was missing on your Simulation Preparation Tool.

Safety & Infection Control
 	
Protect client from injury (i.e., falls, electrical hazards). Follow institution's policy regarding restraints and safety devices.
	Safety—What Is Wrong With This Room?
	
	(Prepare a room in the simulation lab with safety concerns for a client.)
	
	2. Have the students identify what is wrong in the room for an elderly client on suicide precautions (i.e., clutter on the floor, manikin with pierced earrings, restraints are incorrect, equipment with cords, eating utensils left in room, malfunctioning bed alarms, etc.).
	
	   a. List the safety concerns for the client based on their age and clinical condition.
	
	   b. Determine corrective actions.
		Safety—What Is Wrong With This Room?
		
		2. Determine what is wrong in the room for an elderly client on suicide precautions.
		
		   a. List the safety concerns for the client based on age and clinical conditions.
		
		   b. Determine corrective actions.

Evaluating Clinical Performance

IN THIS CHAPTER YOU WILL LEARN ABOUT:

➛ Establishing criteria for clinical evaluation

➛ Providing effective feedback

➛ Implementing the evaluation and documentation process

One of the most challenging aspects of being a clinical instructor is how to be effective in the evaluation of students. You have the responsibility of evaluating whether the student is able to give safe and effective care at their current clinical level and is able to move forward to the next semester or to graduation. This is a huge responsibility. In this chapter we will describe the process of creating an environment conducive for positive and effective evaluation of students' clinical performance.

Evaluation is the ongoing process of observing, comparing, contrasting, and judging students' progress toward achievement of clinical performance outcomes. Students need to know what evaluation criteria will be used and what the consequences will be if they do not meet the criteria (Koharchnik, Weideman, Walters, & Hardy, (2015). Effective evaluation will:

✦ Improve clinical competencies and behaviors.

✦ Motivate student development toward excellence.

✦ Achieve student learning outcomes.

ESTABLISHING CRITERIA FOR CLINICAL EVALUATION

The first step is to determine expectations and student clinical learning outcomes based on course objectives. The course syllabus must define the expected student clinical learning outcomes with clear, measurable evaluation criteria. There are two levels of evaluation that are ongoing in clinical evaluation. These decisions concerning evaluation criteria need to be made by your faculty team and be clearly outlined in the syllabus or the student handbook. Students must be held accountable for meeting clinical learning outcomes.

Another area requiring evaluation is student behaviors. Your syllabus or handbook must define students' behavior that violates current practice and patient safety standards. These should include but are not limited to:

✦ Failure to follow the 7 Rights of Medication Administration.

✦ Number and nature of medication errors allowed as part of the learning process.

✦ Failure to follow infection control standards.

✦ Failure to follow patient safety standards.

✦ Failure to adhere to HIPPA laws.

✦ Failure to communicate important clinical information to the clinical instructor or nursing staff during and at the end of shift.

✦ Failure to document nursing assessments, interventions, evaluation of care.

✦ Perform nursing actions without supervision when supervision is required.

✦ Action or event that could result in harm or death of a client.

Criteria also need to include expectations for attendance, tardiness, and professional behaviors and attire. Other clinical expectations as outlined in Chapter 2 also serve as guidelines for evaluation.

PROVIDING EFFECTIVE FEEDBACK

Timely feedback is an expectation for clinical instructors (Koharchnik, Weideman, Walters, & Hardy (2015). Timely feedback is powerful and provides students information on their strengths and weaknesses. Feedback helps to define for students the expectations on what they need to do each week to meet the clinical learning outcomes.

The concern about giving positive feedback in clinical is shared by many clinical instructors. Instructors are afraid that if they give positive feedback when there are still many things the student needs to do better that they will be sending the message that the student does not need to improve. LET GO OF THAT CONCERN! Positive feedback is so much more powerful than negative feedback. The challenge is to isolate the action the student is doing correctly from the action they need to improve.

Constructive feedback (often perceived as negative feedback) is difficult for most clinical instructors because it is often laden with emotion. It is essential for you as the clinical instructor to be able to transform what may be perceived as negative feedback into constructive feedback that maintains the students' self-esteem. It is important that both positive and constructive feedback be given in a timely manner to reinforce positive behavior and to correct the inappropriate actions before they become habits. Ongoing feedback creates a trusting partnership between the faculty and the student. It is no longer acceptable to give feedback only at midterm and the final because this creates anxiety, fosters lack of trust, and does not provide support for student learning and success (Koharchnik, Weideman, Walters, & Hardy (2015).

Here are some important elements of feedback:

+ Be specific about behaviors observed.

+ Describe who, what, when, where and how.

+ Be timely.

+ Give in private; never in front of others.

+ Use "I" statements to relate your reactions.

The following "Pitfalls" illustrate what NOT to do! When you were a student, you may have experienced some of these negative strategies from your clinical instructor.

+ No news is good news
  Pitfall: Students think they are doing well or they are not doing anything well

+ Negative body language like "The Look" or pointing at the student
  Pitfall: Students think you are angry but they do not know why or are afraid of you

+ The Snapback—responding immediately without thinking in a harsh tone
  Pitfall: Students become intimidated and you look out of control

+ Judgmental
  Pitfall: Destroys the student's self-esteem and is not objective

Feedback is also ineffective and unacceptable when clinical instructors express themselves in highly emotional terms or make dire predictions of consequences like, "If you do not do better, you will never be a good nurse" or "You are not going to pass this clinical if you do not improve." It is *Never Ever* acceptable to call the student stupid or even to insinuate they are dumb or any other negative connotation towards the student. Any of these statements are considered bullying and can destroy the trust you have with the students. Emotional or demeaning statements will result in their loss of respect for you and may put your employment as a clinical instructor in jeopardy.

Feedback requires judgment by the clinical instructor. Here are two examples of a student failing to meet the expectation of being prepared for clinical that have two different outcomes.

EXPECTATION: STUDENTS COME PREPARED FOR CLINICAL

Example 1:

> A student comes unprepared to clinical and states, "I was unable to find the information on my medications I am to give today."
>
> *Instructor Action:* The student should be sent home and receive a written counseling statement if it is the first occurrence. If it is the second occurrence, give a written counseling statement and a clinical day failure.
>
> *Rationale:* This constitutes an unsafe care environment for the client and the student failed to meet a basic expectation outlined in the syllabus for clinical.

Example 2:

> Student says, "I was unable to find the information on my drugs I am to give today. I looked in my medication book and searched the web. This morning I plan to call pharmacy to get the information on the drug."
>
> *Instructor Action:* Give positive feedback.
>
> *Rationale:* The student's action represents information searching and problem solving, both excellent clinical reasoning attributes.

IMPLEMENTING THE DOCUMENTATION AND EVALUATION PROCESS

The concept map provides a valuable tool for you to use in teaching and evaluating the students' progress in clinical. What students write on their concept map is an external representation of their thinking. The most important aspect of the concept map is that you can see the progression of their thinking and the development of their clinical judgment. The concept map is an evolving document that changes as client conditions change and as students improve their ability to provide appropriate care and make clinical judgments. Below are some tips for using the concept map as an evaluation tool.

+ The value of requiring a concept map before clinical is to assure students are safe and are prepared for clinical.

+ It is impossible for the concept map to be 100% correct before the student has assessed the client.

✦ The emphasis on evaluation and/or grading the concept map should be placed on the student's ability to make changes based on their assessment of the client, the client's response to the care, and evaluation and judgment about the care given.

The clinical instructor knows the student is becoming more sophisticated in their clinical reasoning when they are able to evaluate and use clinical judgment to make decisions about what care is needed in the future. A rubric that can be used to grade the concept map can be found in Chapter 4.

As we stated earlier, evaluation is an ongoing process. As a clinical instructor, look for trends in the students' clinical performance. Timely feedback and weekly evaluations are essential to identify the trends. The advantages of weekly evaluations are that they provide:

✦ Trends: positive or negative.

✦ Documentation of performance.

✦ Timely feedback.

✦ Motivate student development.

✦ Assist clinical instructors with clinical assignments.

Evaluation requires a tool that accurately reflects clinical learning outcomes that are standards-based and meet course outcomes. The tool should list the specific criteria necessary for students to meet the learning outcomes. In other words, do your evaluation criteria measure what you want your students to achieve? A well-constructed evaluation tool should be used weekly, at mid-term and for the final evaluation (Refer to Appendix A—Clinical Evaluation Tool).

Appendix A, **Clinical Evaluation Tool**, reflects the SAFETY model (Refer to Chapter 8), nursing process, practice, safety, and NCLEX® standards, clinical application of key NCLEX® standards, professional behaviors, and required written clinical care plans and concept maps. The course syllabus should include: the process for clinical evaluation, when counseling is necessary, what constitutes a clinical day failure, and when clinical day failures result in course failure (Refer to Appendix B—Example of Policies for the Course Syllabus).

Anecdotal notes are an excellent supplement to the weekly evaluation tool (Koharchnik, Weideman, Walters, & Hardy, 2015). These are the personal property of the clinical instructor and include information not on the weekly evaluation tool. They are not part of the permanent record unless the clinical instructor makes them available to others. Good anecdotal notes are the story behind your observations, a way to capture your thoughts, or the message your "gut" is giving you. We have all had moments in clinical with a student where the red flag went up but you just could not put your finger on it. The anecdotal notes are the place to write the objective information surrounding that event. They provide a more detailed account of the student's clinical performance that day. In addition, they can serve as excellent backup documentation when a student should have a clinical day failure (Refer to Appendix C—Example of Anecdotal Notes).

Weekly evaluation of the student provides you the necessary information about the student's progress and the trends become evident. Questions to ask yourself:

+ Is the student receiving "satisfactory" every week and making acceptable progress?

+ Is the student receiving some "needs improvement" in certain areas but you observe progress in the area the next week?

Action: None needed, continue to evaluate and document student's progress.

BUT:

+ Is the student receiving "needs improvement" or "unsatisfactory" in the same areas over a number of weeks with no progress?

Action: Counseling session needed.

Counseling serves to formally notify the student their performance is unsatisfactory. There are two levels of counseling:

+ The counseling session identifies needed actions or behaviors to progress and includes consequences if the student does not improve.

+ The counseling session identifies a significant event or action that resulted in, or potentially could have resulted in, client harm and the ensuing consequences, i.e., clinical day failure or course failure.

Use Appendix D, Guide for Clinical Evaluation, to assist in your decision to counsel a student and to decide, if needed, the level of consequences for the incident. It is important to the success of your student that you are able to determine when the situation requires counseling and when it is a teaching moment. Teaching moments are powerful tools and can often be done immediately. It is also the opportunity to refer students back to their references, or they may need a day in the lab or simulation to refresh essential clinical competencies.

If counseling or documentation of the situation is needed, we recommend using the "STAR" format for counseling. This is a concise format, easy to use and keeps both clinical instructors and students focused on the facts of the situation (Refer to Appendix E– STAR Counseling Form).

STAR

S = Situation: Describe the situation.

T = Task: What was supposed to be accomplished, or what were the requirements, standards of practice or policies that were not met? Include standards or policies as appropriate.

A = Action: Plan for Action: What does the student need to do to improve?

Consequences: What are the consequences if corrective action is not met? A time frame for improvement must be stated.

R = Results: Follow-up sessions: Were actions accomplished? What was the outcome?

Two examples of completed **STAR Counseling Forms** are included for your reference (Refer to Appendix F–Example STAR Counseling Form and Appendix G–Example STAR Counseling Warning/Unsatisfactory Course Performance/Clinical Day Failure Form).

Clinical instructors worry about an unsafe event that occurs on the last day of clinical. Does the event warrant failing the student? Remember, an unsafe event that occurs on the first or the last day of clinical requires action. By following a well-written and implemented evaluation process on a weekly basis, the clinical instructor will have the documentation needed to fail the student from clinical and/or the course depending on what constitutes failure.

STEPS FOR EFFECTIVE COUNSELING

When you decide a counseling session is necessary, we recommend the following steps:

- ✦ Inform the student you are concerned about their clinical performance and that you will notify them when the counseling session will occur. (DO NOT make hasty decisions you may regret or cannot support. Consult the course coordinator.)

- ✦ Complete the STAR counseling form (be objective and stick to the facts). You may need to include observations from an earlier time with the specific incident and date that you included in your anecdotal notes.

- ✦ Have the course coordinator or other neutral party review the counseling statement for clarity, appropriate steps and consequences prior to the session.

- ✦ Notify the student and the witness of the scheduled counseling time.

- ✦ Set the structure for the counseling session with the student when they arrive: purpose of the meeting, introduce the witness, and begin with the situation as written on the counseling form.

- ✦ Be prepared to move the discussion back to the focus of the counseling session if the student wants to deviate to other topics.

- ✦ If the student becomes too emotional, recognize the emotion, give the student time to collect their thoughts, and if needed, give them a break.

- ✦ When you are done presenting the situation, give the student an opportunity to express their side of the story. (Note: there is a place on the form for the student to write their comments.)

- ✦ After the student presents their side of the story, proceed as planned or if the student brings new information to the situation that may change actions or consequences, inform the student that you will reassess the new information and will reschedule another counseling session.

- ✦ At the conclusion of the session, the student signs the form. If the student refuses to sign the form, let them know the signature only indicates they have seen the form and the session occurred. They can write in the comment section if they disagree. If the student still refuses to sign, just note that on the counseling form.

- ✦ Other signatures include yours and the witness. Be sure it is dated and timed.

- ✦ A copy is given to the student.

- ✦ REMAIN CALM AT ALL TIMES!!!!!!

Regardless of what your counseling and evaluation processes are, they need to be reviewed by your college or university legal team. Luckily these situations, although extremely distressing, happen infrequently. Most of the time, the evaluation process is positive. The students improve their skills and abilities; are motivated for future growth; and, best of all, they are successful in achieving the clinical learning outcomes.

CLINICAL EVALUATION TOOL

Chapter 7

Clinical Evaluation Tool Using "SAFETY" Model

Student Name:

Clinical Date:

PERFORMANCE OUTCOMES	Mid-Term																Final			
	S	NI	U	S	NI	U	S	NI	U	S	NI	U	S	NI	U	NA	S	NI	U	NA
Prepared for all facets of clinical day, (care based on SAFETY (i.e., patho, asses, labs, diag tests, interventions, skills, meds, etc).																				
System-Specific Assessment																				
Performs system-specific assessments based on pathophysiology of disease & client need; reports/documents, assessments.																				
Reports/documents clinical findings; Recognizes deviations from client's normal.																				
Reviews & reports lab / diagnostic test findings that deviate from normal																				
Analysis: Concepts/ Outcomes																				
Analysis of concepts, desired outcomes appropriate & measureable based on assessment findings.																				
Idenitfies if client condition is acute/chronic.																				
First-Do Priority Interventions																				
Plans & prioritizes delivery of care/orders (interventions).																				
Perform/document invasive nursing procedures with supervision only.																				
Sterile procedure/ standard of care followed.																				
Medication protocol/preparation/administration/ documentation (i.e., *Checks MAR against orders *Prepares/calculates dosage appropriately *Has needed data (i.e., VS, labs, etc.).																				

177

Page 1

CLINICAL EVALUATION TOOL *(cont'd)*

Student Name:

Clinical Date:

Clinical Evaluation Tool Using "SAFETY" Model

	Mid-Term																		Final			
PERFORMANCE OUTCOMES	S	NI	U	S	NI	U	S	NI	U	S	NI	U	S	NI	U	NA	S	NI	U	S	NI	U	NA
Identifies client x 2 with every medication administered.																							
Administers medications under supervision of instructor; Never administer; Sub cu, IV, IM, nasal gastric, peg without instructor.																							
Evaluation of Outcomes																							
Evaluation of progress toward desired outcomes.																							
Makes changes in plan of care as appropriate.																							
Evaluates medications for desired outcomes, undesirable effects, interactions, complications.																							
Assess if progress toward outcomes is being met; makes changes as appropriate.																							
Trend for Potential Complications																							
Seeks guidance as appropriate.																							
Notifies instructor/nurse re: trends /changes in client condition, complications with meds and/or post-procedure & intervene as appropriate.																							
Yes- You Manage Care to Reduce "RISKS"																							
Discuss appropriate management activities to include: delegation, room assign, equipment safety, etc. for specific client's needs.																							
Maintains client safety (fall prevention, bed position, call light, infection control, equipment etc).																							

CLINICAL EVALUATION TOOL (cont'd)

Student Name:

Clinical Date:

Clinical Evaluation Tool Using "SAFETY" Model

PERFORMANCE OUTCOMES	Mid-Term																		Final		
	S	NI	U	S	NI	U	S	NI	U	S	NI	U	S	NI	U	S	NI	U	NA	S	NI	U	NA	S	NI	U	S	NI	U	S	NI	U	S	NI	U	S	NI	U	NA
Communication																					
Written & computer charting complete, timely & cosigned by end of shift. Demonstrates ability to use Inform systems technology.																					
Uses theraupeutic communication techniques.																					
Non-verbal communication: Aware of importance & impact.																					
Gives concise, accurate, complete report at end of day following SBAR before leaving assigned unit.																					
Client teaching concise, accurate; includes health promotion & plan for transitional care.																					
Professional Behavior																					
Integrates standards of care, scope of practice, ethical & cultural practice into client care.																					
Coordinates/colloborates/advocates with interdisciplinary team.																					
Accepts constructive criticism.																					
Maintains client/institutional confidentiality i.e., HIPAA.																					
Assertive in seeking learning experiences.																					
Respectful of clients personnel; manages conflict.																					
Reports on time to unit/conferences & uses spare time constructively.																					
Adheres to Core Values / handbook/syllabus.																					
Follow school dress code as outlined in handbook/syllabus.																					

APPENDIX A

Chapter 7

CLINICAL EVALUATION TOOL *(cont'd)*

Student Name: _____

Clinical Date: _____

Clinical Evaluation Tool Using "SAFETY" Model

PERFORMANCE OUTCOMES													Mid-Term												Final			
	S	NI	U	S	NI	U	S	NI	U	S	NI	U	S	NI	U	NA	S	NI	U	S	NI	U	S	NI	U	S	NI	U	NA
Concept Map																													
Written concept map, w/system-spec assess, priority interventions, eval. of client response & progress toward outcomes, patho page, 2 AIDES sheets & Reflection Questions.																													
Paperwork turned in on time.																													
Faculty/student initials																													

S: Satisfactory; NI: Needs Improvement; U: Unsatisfactory; NA: Not experienced

S: Clinical behavior is safe & demonstrates growth toward course competencies.

NI: Clinical behavior is safe, however, performance is deficient in essential background knowledge.

U: Clinical behavior is unsafe. Performance seldom demonstrates essential knowledge & growth toward competencies.

NA: Clinical behavior not relevant to assigned client.

Absences _____ Late arrivals _____

Final Clinical Grade _____

Faculty _____ Date _____

Student _____ Date _____

Comments:

EXAMPLE OF POLICIES FOR A SYLLABUS

CLINICAL PRACTICE ATTENDANCE POLICY

▲ *Students are expected to attend all clinical activities, including simulation lab and extrinsic sites.* Absences will be considered only if certified as unavoidable because of sickness or other causes, such as accident or death of immediate family member, and student provides documentation (such as doctor's excuse for illness, etc.).

▲ **Unexcused clinical absences will result in a clinical day failure for each missed clinical experience.**

▲ **Two clinical day failures will result in a course failure.** For example, unacceptable reasons for missing a clinical experience are work, travel, or social reasons.

▲ Make-up time for missed clinical nursing experiences will be **determined at the discretion of the course coordinator and availability of clinical facilities** and lab facilities.

▲ Failure to complete make up clinical may result in course failure.

▲ **A student will notify their clinical instructor verbally at least 1 hour prior to the absence and notify the course coordinator within 24 hours. Faculty may require withdrawal of any student who has missed sufficient clinical to prevent completion of clinical objectives.**

CLINICAL EXPECTATIONS

It is expected that students in a professional nursing program will be **consistently on time and prepared** for all lab, clinical, and simulation assignments.

Any student reporting unprepared, no equipment, inappropriately dressed or not completing clinical preparation prior to lab, clinical, and simulation or any other non-professional behavior will:

▲ 1st offense = student will receive a warning and receive a written counseling statement.

▲ 2nd offense = student will be sent home with Clinical Day Failure and receive a written counseling statement.

▲ 3rd offense = student will be sent home and receive a Clinical Day Failure which will constitute a course failure.

TARDINESS POLICY:

Late arrival to clinical, simulation, or post-conference is not acceptable. Any student reporting to clinical or the lab late after the scheduled time (as scheduled weekly) is subject to penalties and consequences associated with professionalism and accountability.

▲ For the 1st offense = student will receive a verbal warning with a written counseling statement.

▲ For the 2nd offense = student will be sent home and receive a Clinical Day Failure with a written counseling statement.

▲ For a 3rd offense = student will be sent home and receive a Clinical Day Failure which will constitute a course failure.

APPENDIX C

EXAMPLE OF ANECDOTAL NOTES

9/2	Did not receive clinical assignment. Attempted to contact student at both contact numbers provided by the student. Was unable to reach student or leave a message at either number. Course coordinator aware of this and present during phone attempts.
9/7	Discussed assignment not received and inability to leave messages. Student stated they were out of town and has had phone and computer troubles. Turned in hard copy of assignment. Discussed the importance of timeliness of clinical work.
9/14	Student turned in assignment on time on 9/9, but had used the previous week's questions; she was unaware of the updated assignment. Discussed the need to ensure she checks for the updated assignments.
9/16	Student did not turn in assignment related to hyperbarics experience.
9/21	Student stated she was "unaware there was an assignment associated with this." She e-mailed it that evening.
	Counseled student regarding the late and inaccurate assignments. Explained so far her clinical performance was very good, but she needs to be organized and aware of deadlines and must meet these as assigned. I asked her to think about what she could do to improve her behaviors. She stated she "has a lot going on," but would make every effort to do so. She said poor organization is a weakness of hers.
	Discussed this with course coordinator and was instructed to continue to document interactions and discussions.
9/28	Absent—was called the prior night and informed that she would be out because her daughter had an ear infection. Course coordinator notified.
11/9	Absent—contacted the night prior. Student stated she had a virus. (The next time we spoke, 11/12, student stated by clinical morning she had felt better, but her son then had the virus.)
11/16	Confirmed make-up day for 11/14 and asked about excuse. She stated she would get one as requested by course coordinator. She stated she was not given a deadline for this.
11/22	I contacted student via e-mail to let her know I had not received her ED extrinsic assignment. Student contacted me by phone that evening to let me know she had sent it that day after receiving my e-mail and must have forgotten to send it when she completed it last week.
	I then read her e-mail, see attached, and had to contact her again because the assignment was not attached to the e-mail. Student said she had printed a copy and would bring it to clinical the following day.
	Contacted course coordinator to discuss student's late assignments and absences for direction on how to proceed. Both assignments were pass/fail. Coordinator advised since they were turned in complete, they should be considered passing.
11/23	Student turned in hard copy of ED extrinsic.
11/24	Make up clinical day

GUIDE FOR CLINICAL EVALUATION
VERY IMPORTANT TO EVALUATE EACH INCIDENT SEPARATELY
Requires faculty professional judgment
Look for patterns, trends in behavior

DIRECTIONS: THIS GUIDE SHOULD BE ADAPTED

▲ Per your curriculum and level of students.

▲ Per your State Board of Nursing guidelines for students and faculty in clinical.

▲ Per your school or college guidelines, process for reviewing patterns and trends for behavior of students.

▲ Based on faculty, definitions of what constitutes *client safety*, *professional issues*, *clinical day failure*, and *course failure* should be included in the course syllabus.

▲ Note: For any concerns or questions about patterns or trends in a student's behavior, consult with your course coordinator and/or faculty team. (Always good to keep anecdotal notes on students when there are issues.)

STUDENT PROFESSIONAL OR CLINICAL ISSUE

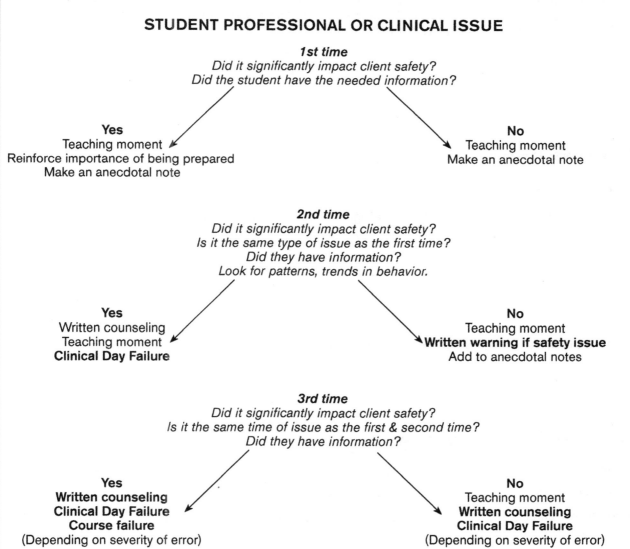

1st time
Did it significantly impact client safety?
Did the student have the needed information?

Yes
Teaching moment
Reinforce importance of being prepared
Make an anecdotal note

No
Teaching moment
Make an anecdotal note

2nd time
Did it significantly impact client safety?
Is it the same type of issue as the first time?
Did they have information?
Look for patterns, trends in behavior.

Yes
Written counseling
Teaching moment
Clinical Day Failure

No
Teaching moment
Written warning if safety issue
Add to anecdotal notes

3rd time
Did it significantly impact client safety?
Is it the same time of issue as the first & second time?
Did they have information?

Yes
Written counseling
Clinical Day Failure
Course failure
(Depending on severity of error)

No
Teaching moment
Written counseling
Clinical Day Failure
(Depending on severity of error)

APPENDIX E

STAR COUNSELING FORM

Faculty Name: _____

Date of Incident: _____

Student Name: _____

Date of Session: _____

S – SITUATION: Describe the situation.

T – TASK: Requirements and/or policy performance standards that are not being met. (Standards and evaluation criteria published in course syllabus and/or in the University or College of Nursing student handbooks). State reference with page number(s) if applicable.

A – ACTIONS: Plan to improve unsatisfactory performance.

Consequences: Consequences of not meeting performance improvement plan.

R – RESULTS: Date: (Results from actions listed above)

DATE TO IMPROVE PERFORMANCE BY:

Faculty Signature: _____   Date: _____

Student Signature: _____   Date: _____

Observer Signature: _____   Date: _____

APPENDIX F

EXAMPLE STAR COUNSELING FORM

Faculty Name: <u>Professor Clinical</u>   Date of Incident: <u>January 12, 2017</u>

Student Name: <u>Minnie Student</u>   Date of Session: <u>January 17, 2017</u>

S – SITUATION: Describe the situation:

1. Wore brown shoes to clinical. Stated it was because she had washed her shoes and they were not dry.
2. When asked where her stethoscope was, as she was getting ready for her assessment, she reported it was in the conference room.
3. Conducted an equipment check at the end of clinical and she did not have stethoscope or watch.

T – TASK: Requirements and/or policy performance standards that are not being met. (Safety standards and evaluation criteria published in course syllabus.) State reference with page number(s).

Reference: Course Syllabus. Page 8: Clinical Preparation & Dress Code

Page 11: Statement of Academic Responsibility and clinical orientation

Evaluation Criteria: Ethical behavior

A – ACTIONS: Steps to be taken to improve unsatisfactory performance:

1. Come to clinical in appropriate clinical uniform with white shoes.
2. Bring all equipment needed, stethoscope, watch, scissors, and protective eyewear.
3. Answer questions honestly.

Consequences: Consequences of not meeting performance improvement plan:

Failure to wear correct uniform and bring equipment to clinical will result in being sent home from clinical with a clinical day failure.

Date to improve performance by: Begin immediately with next clinical day, January 19, 2017

Faculty Signature: *Professor Clinical*   Student Signature: *Minnie Student*

Observer Signature: *Professor Lab*

R – RESULTS: Date: (Results from action listed above)

1. Came appropriately dressed for clinical.
2. Had equipment needed for clinical.
3. No further incidents of dishonesty.

FURTHER ACTION NEEDED (none, further counseling, consequences imposed):

No further action needed

Faculty Signature: *Professor Clinical*   Student Signature: *Minnie Student*

Observer Signature: *Professor Lab*

APPENDIX G

EXAMPLE STAR COUNSELING WARNING/UNSATISFACTORY COURSE PERFORMANCE/CLINICAL DAY FAILURE FORM

Faculty Name: _____ Student Name: _____

Date of Counseling Session: <u>January 17, 2017</u> Date of Incident: <u>January 12, 2017</u>

S – SITUATION: Describe the situation. Course requirement not being met:

Gave Oxycodone, a narcotic, to her client without the knowledge or supervision of the clinical faculty. (Reference: Number 6 under Medication Error Policy, page 10 of 323 Syllabus)

1. Could not answer questions about the actions of the medication. (Reference: Number 6 under Medication Error Policy, page 10 of 323 Syllabus)
2. Medication was not signed out, count was not done and no documentation of the medication was given. (Reference Number 5 under Medication Error Policy, page 10 of syllabus)
3. The client was not assessed for level or type of pain. Client's husband requested the pain medication for his wife. (Reference Number 5 under Medication Error Policy, page 10 of syllabus)

T – TASK: Requirements and/or policy performance standards that are not being met:

Reference: (Reference: Number 6 under Medication Error Policy, page 10 of Syllabus)

Student Medication Error Policy, page 10 of the Course Syllabus

Guidelines for clinical performance given in orientation for clinical on January 5, 2017

A – ACTIONS: Steps taken to improve unsatisfactory performance:

1. All medications will be given under the supervision of your clinical faculty until you are notified otherwise.
2. Know the action and significant side effects of all medications prior to administering the medication.
3. All medications need to be correctly documented per hospital policy.
4. Failure to do so will result in a 2nd clinical day failure.

R – RESULTS: Date: Pending (Results from action listed above)

DATE TO IMPROVE PERFORMANCE BY: Immediately beginning with the next clinical day on January 19, 2017.

Faculty Signature: _____ Date: _____

Student Signature: _____ Date: _____

Observer Signature: _____ Date: _____

To be filed: Faculty files, Student file in Student Services

ENGAGING THE LEARNER ACTIVITIES

STUDENT-CENTERED LEARNING ACTIVITIES
LINKED TO PROFESSIONAL AND NCLEX® STANDARDS

Resources Needed for Activity	The Eight-Step Approach for Teaching Clinical Nursing (Zager, Manning & Herman, 2017)	The Eight-Step Approach for Student Clinical Success (Zager, Manning & Herman, 2017)
Standards	**Faculty Instructions**	**Student Instructions**

Psychosocial Integrity
 	
Manage conflict among clients and healthcare staff.
 	
Physiological Integrity; Basic Care
 	
Monitor client's hydration status.
	Professional Behavior: Conflict Management
	(Refer to Appendix A)
	
	Activity is based on the Clinical Evaluation Tool, Professional Behaviors, Managing conflict. *Have students work in pairs.*
	
	1. Present each pair of students with a brief scenario of a conflict between students about the care of a client with fluid volume deficit.
	
	  a. 1st student assesses VS and finds the VS are not within normal range, does not report it, and wants to check VS again in an hour.
	
	  b. 2nd student wants to report the abnormal VS now because it is the expectation to report changes in VS's and it could be a potential complication of fluid volume deficit.
	
	  c. Have the students answer the questions:
	
	    1). What is the standard of practice?
	
	    2). What are the potential complications based on the assessed VS and the client's diagnosis (i.e. fluid volume deficit)?
	
	    3). Determine the steps to take when they disagree with their colleague on the plan of care (i.e. offer to re-check the VS or ask the nurse or instructor, etc.).
	
	    4). What happens if they take no action?
	
	    5). What happens if the 2nd student reports the VS even if the 1st student does not agree?
	
	  d. What is the most appropriate decision?
		Professional Behavior: Conflict Management
		(Refer to end of Chapter 7, Clinical Evaluation Tool)
		
		Work with a partner.
		
		1. Your client has a fluid volume imbalance.
		
		  a. 1st student assess the VS and notes VS are not within normal range. You want to check the VS again in an hour instead of reporting the change now.
		
		  b. 2nd student you want to report the abnormal VS now because the expectation is to report changes in VS's to the nurse and/or instructor. You are concerned about potential complications.
		
		  c. Answer the questions:
		
		    1). What are the practice standards?
		
		    2). What are the potential complications based on the assessed VS and the client's diagnosis?
		
		    3). What steps could you take when you disagree with your colleague on the plan of care?
		
		    4). What happens if you take no action?
		
		    5). What happens if the 2nd student reports the VS even if the 1st student does not agree?
		
		  d. What is the most appropriate decision?

NOTES

Linking Clinical Experience to NCLEX® Success

IN THIS CHAPTER YOU WILL LEARN HOW TO:

→ Apply NCLEX® standards throughout the clinical experience

→ Adapt structures organized from the NCLEX® standards to assist in mastering clinical reasoning

APPLY NCLEX® STANDARDS THROUGHOUT THE CLINICAL EXPERIENCE

As a clinical instructor, you are one of the most important and powerful professionals in preparing the student nurse for both clinical and NCLEX® success. Now that you have reviewed the chapters in this book, from how to start teaching clinical to evaluating the clinical experience, let's move on to strategies for incorporating NCLEX® standards throughout the clinical experience.

The purpose of the NCLEX-RN® is to ensure public protection. The exam evaluates specific competencies necessary for the newly licensed, entry-level registered nurse to perform safe and effective care. The NCLEX-RN® Test Plan provides an abbreviated summary of the content and scope of the licensing examination. This plan is currently revised every three years. The Test Plan can be downloaded from the National Council State Board of Nursing's website (www.ncsbn.org). It provides a compass for preparation of the nursing student to perform successful clinical practice.

Unfortunately many clinical faculty report feeling overwhelmed by being held accountable for their students' success on the NCLEX®. There is a sense of urgency for faculty to teach everything to the nursing students, when in reality this creates a sense of chaos for both the student and the faculty member. Since you are reading this book and have made it to this chapter, we are confident that you, too, may share some of these similar feelings. The good news is there are strategies to assist you in simplifying this overwhelming sense of responsibility while at the same time increasing both clinical and NCLEX® success for your students.

Incorporating and linking these activities, as outlined in the current NCLEX-RN® Test Plan, to the clinical experience is a very powerful strategy to ensure the students have an appropriate focus during their clinical experience. For example, whether the student is in medical-surgical, intensive care, obstetrics, or pediatric clinical, the clinical objectives and evaluation tools should reflect the NCLEX® Activity Statements. In addition to clinical, these same activities need to be incorporated throughout the classroom presentations and examination items.

In order to prioritize these activities, we have organized these within the framework of three mnemonics—"SAFETY", "RISK", and "AIDES"—to provide structures for organizing priority NCLEX® activities. (Refer to Appendix A–"SAFETY", Appendix B–"RISK", and Appendix C–"AIDES".)

ADAPT STRUCTURES ORGANIZED FROM THE NCLEX® STANDARDS

Some examples of how you may adapt the mnemonic "SAFETY" to linking the clinical experience to NCLEX® success begins with reviewing the letters beginning with the S in "SAFETY". The S represents both **System-Specific Physiology** and **System-Specific Assessments**. System-Specific Physiology does not matter what clinical rotation the student is in, the student must be taught to develop an understanding of what is physiologically taking place with the client. As the student is just beginning clinical, it may be sufficient for the student to understand the reason a school-age child experiences frequent swallowing after a tonsillectomy is due to bleeding. After the student understands this physiological change, then the student needs to begin to understand the pathophysiology regarding the changes in the heart rate, respiratory rate, blood pressure, skin color and temperature, and urine output that can occur if the bleeding is not evaluated initially and an early intervention is not implemented. This is a great opportunity for you to take advantage of the teaching moment and compare these vital sign changes and assist the student in making links and connections.

As the student grows and develops throughout the curriculum, the student needs to also begin to compare and contrast the similarities/differences in the physiology/pathophysiology between adults and children.

With this teaching strategy, the following NCLEX® activities are reviewed:

✔ Identify pathophysiology related to an acute or chronic condition (i.e., signs and symptoms).

✔ Assess and respond to changes in vital signs.

System-Specific Assessment, part of the S in "SAFETY", is another example of how clinical experience can be linked to NCLEX® success. No matter what clinical rotation the student is in, the student must be taught how to complete a fast system-specific assessment with a focus on the presenting symptoms versus a detailed one-hour head-to-toe assessment. The students must learn to master the process of assessing from the minute they walk into the client's room. When they come to clinical, students do not have this cognitive skill unless it is taught in every unit and practiced every clinical day. If the students are in the pediatric clinical rotation and the school-age child is bleeding after a tonsillectomy, then this is an excellent opportunity to assist students in understanding that the unique system-specific assessment is the frequent swallowing and recognize the vital sign changes for the specific child's developmental stage. After this has been reviewed, then compare these vital sign changes to the various developmental stages and/or even the vital signs for an adult.

As a clinical instructor, you have another opportunity to assist the student in connecting the similarities and/or differences in both the system-specific assessments and the TRENDS with the hemodynamic changes that may occur with any client who is bleeding. Teaching trending is important, so the student learns the early versus the late signs and symptoms for hemorrhaging. Reviewing signs and symptoms of bleeding without organizing these around early versus late signs does not facilitate the ongoing development of clinical reasoning. Every clinical experience is an opportunity to assist students in learning how to master the skill of clinical reasoning.

As the student progresses throughout the curriculum, it is important for the clinical instructor to assist students in reviewing the **differences** between the system-specific assessments for a client who is bleeding post-op GI surgery, post-cardiac catheterization, fracture, placenta previa, abruption placenta, etc. It is also important for the student to recognize the **similarities** between the hemodynamic changes that occur with any client who is bleeding. It goes without saying, that it is imperative to review the appropriate nursing interventions for the child who is bleeding following a tonsillectomy as well as comparing the differences/similarities in the nursing care for other clients who are bleeding for various reasons. This will be discussed further with the **F** in "SAFETY". Four additional NCLEX® activities have now been discussed under system-specific assessments:

- ✔ Perform focused assessment and re-assessment.

- ✔ Assess and respond to changes in vital signs.

- ✔ Recognize signs and symptoms of complications and intervene appropriately when providing care.

- ✔ Recognize trends and changes in client condition and intervene.

It is imperative that students learn to master the habit of reviewing "**System-specific labs and diagnostic procedures**" through analyzing lab values and performing diagnostic tests (i.e., EKG, O_2 saturation, glucose monitoring, etc.). There is an emphasis on diagnostic tests and procedures under the Client Need Category of Reduction of Risk on the NCLEX–RN®. During each clinical experience, the students should develop the habit of reviewing lab values and linking the significance of these to their client's nursing care. In order to provide both you and your students with a structure for this, we have included a **Lab & Diagnostic Tests and Procedures Tool** in Chapter 4, Appendix H. (Specific information regarding these can be reviewed in the book *Nursing Made Insanely Easy* by Manning & Rayfield, 2016.) This process has addressed the following NCLEX® activities:

D iagnostic test results—monitor; intervene for complications.

I njury and/or complications from procedure should be prevented.

A ssist with invasive procedures (e.g., thoracentesis, bronchoscopy).

G lucose monitoring, ECG, O_2 saturation, etc. may be performed.

N ote client's response to procedures and treatments.

O btain specimens other than blood (e.g., wound, stool, etc.).

S igns and symptoms of trends and/or changes-monitor, and intervene.

T each client and family about procedures and treatments.

I dentify vital signs and monitor for changes and intervene.

C omplications should be noted and followed immediately with an action.

The **A** in "SAFETY" represents "**Analyzing priority nursing concepts**" based on the system-specific assessments. The nursing student needs to learn how to review and assess several nursing concepts for a specific client in addition to several different clients and prioritize the care for these clients. This is an excellent opportunity for you to assist the student in understanding how to appropriately triage or prioritize nursing care. This can also be a great topic for pre/post conferences. The NCLEX® activity addressed for this process is:

✔ Assess/triage clients to prioritize order of care delivery.

The **F** in "SAFETY" represents both nursing interventions that should be implemented "**First**" as well as medications that should be administered "**First**". When the client has four nursing interventions in need of implementation, then you can assist the student by consistently asking questions such as: *"What are the priority nursing actions? What client needs to be evaluated first and why? Which client needs immediate nursing action and why? What medications should be administered first for specific clinical assessments?"*

For example, if a client begins expectorating blood and the client is positioned in the supine position, then the priority nursing action would be to reposition client even prior to notifying healthcare provider or initiating a complete assessment. If the student has two clients bleeding, then you can facilitate the process of clinical reasoning by reviewing the changes with the trends in the vital signs, I & O, and/or LOC to assist in identifying if the clients are experiencing early or late signs of bleeding.

Another example of how you can assist the student in prioritizing, is if the client has respiratory problems and has an order to administer a corticosteroid inhaler and a Beta$_2$ Adrenergic Agonist such as Albuterol, then you may want to help the student in connecting the actions for both of these drugs with the pathophysiology. This will assist them in understanding the rationale for administering Albuterol prior to the steroid inhaler. This will assist in reviewing the NCLEX® activity:

✔ Prioritize workload to manage time effectively.

The **E** in "SAFETY" will assist the student in always remembering to "Evaluate the "Expected Outcomes" from the nursing care as well as from the medications. These evaluations might include:

✦ Did the bleeding stop?

✦ Did the breath sounds improve?

✦ Did the vital signs return to baseline?

✦ Did the medication assist in reducing the intracranial pressure?

✦ Did the medication assist in reducing the serum glucose?

The NCLEX® activities addressed include:

✔ Evaluate/document response to treatment.

✔ Evaluate therapeutic effect of medications.

"Trend for Potential Complications" in the client's assessment, **T** in "SAFETY," is an excellent observation to determine the client's clinical status. Students must consistently compare and contrast vital signs, I & O, neurological assessments, drainage, etc. (For a complete review of "Trends to monitor for preventing complications", refer to the book *Nursing Made Insanely Easy*, pp. 8-9, Manning & Rayfield, 2016.) As students become more proficient with the trending of the assessment findings, then they need to begin to organize the assessments into early versus late clinical findings. If the client is unstable and presenting with late signs and symptoms, then it is imperative for the student to be competent at intervening with the priority intervention(s) to prevent the client from deteriorating and experiencing a crisis.

For example, if the client begins hemorrhaging two hours post-op, the student needs to assess the subtle changes with the heart rate and respiratory rate elevation and restlessness, and recognize the potential complication with bleeding and the priority nursing interventions prior to the client progressing to hypovolemic shock.

Another example of trends would be if the client was receiving Magnesium Sulfate and the urine output had been 85 mL/hour, and the next hour the urine output is 45 mL/hour. Magnesium Sulfate is excreted in the urine, and with this trend it would be imperative to report this decline and not wait for the urine to continue to decline. The student needs your assistance and support to learn how to develop this clinical judgment. With role-modeling your thinking, this will assist the student to begin understanding this process. This will take a lot of practice, but with your consistent encouragement and assistance, it will become part of the structure for thinking as the student develops and implements the plan of care. The NCLEX® activities represent the Client Need Category of Reduction of Risk and are reviewed below:

✔ Recognize trends and changes in client condition and intervene.

✔ Recognize signs and symptoms of complications and intervene appropriately when providing care.

✔ Assess and respond to changes in vital signs.

The Y in "SAFETY" represents management. **"Yes, Management is important to prevent "RISK" to our clients!"** (Refer to Chapter 3, Appendix A–Quick Approach: Inquiry Questions for Classroom and Clinical Knowledge Organized Around the "SAFETY" Model) for examples of NCLEX® activities reflecting Management and Safety on the NCLEX®. These activities will be useful to connect throughout clinical for both client safety and to assist with NCLEX® success. "RISK" (Appendix B) is a mnemonic that will help the student from day one in clinical, know what to assess for to prevent "RISKS". The assessments include:

✦ Risk for falls

✦ Practice infection control

✦ Identify client correctly

✦ Review accuracy of orders

✦ Assess and prevent skin breakdown

✦ Practice equipment safety

✦ Understand Standards of Practice

✦ Practice effective documentation

✦ Client teaching

The mnemonic "AIDES" is also a structure for organizing the NCLEX® activities that have a focus on pharmacology. This is a great tool to use throughout the curriculum, so the students in clinical know what the expectations are from semester to semester. In many situations, the clinical instructors focus on different aspects of pharmacology, and as soon as the students understand what the instructor wants, it is time for a new clinical rotation. "AIDES" reflect NCLEX® standards, so if these are consistently reviewed based on the student's educational development and level within the curriculum, students will have a better understanding of what it takes to be successful regarding pharmacology on the NCLEX®.

These three mnemonics (Refer to Appendix A–SAFETY, Appendix B–AIDES and Appendix C–RISK) will serve as a compass to you and your students while integrating NCLEX® standards during the clinical experience. Please note that while many of the NCLEX® activities from the NCLEX® Test Plan are represented within the mnemonics, these are not all inclusive. A complete list of these can be downloaded from the National Council of State Boards of Nursing (www. ncbn.org). It is very powerful when we start from Day 1 in clinical, adapting these standards and level these throughout the curriculum. When clinical faculty adapt these throughout each clinical rotation and are consistent with expectations, paperwork, classroom presentations, exam items throughout the curriculum, simulation, and the evaluation process, nursing students have an excellent roadmap for NCLEX® success. These standards can and should be the framework for the various teaching strategies outlined in previous chapters. The **Quick Approach: Inquiry Questions for Clinical Knowledge Organized Around the Nursing Process** (Chapter 3, Appendix A) and the **Clinical Evaluation Tool** (Chapter 7, Appendix A) help link clinical to NCLEX®.

Clinical nursing instructors hold a very powerful key to students' success. It is in the clinical experience where students report they begin making connections from theory to clinical practice. Linking NCLEX® with your clinical teaching and evaluating is indeed the ticket to your students' success.

SAFETY

This structure can help prioritize NCLEX® activities that can be evaluated through the **Concept Map, History and Pathophysiology Information and Reflection Questions** (see Chapter 4 appendixes).

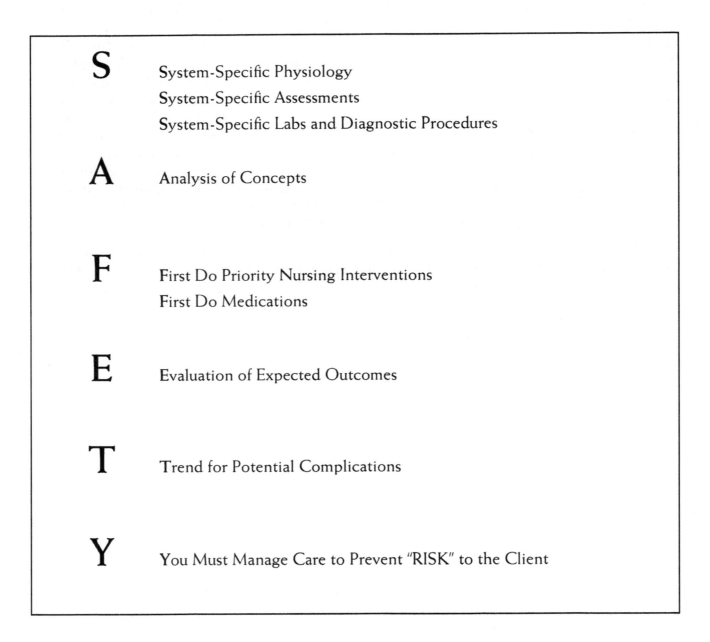

S
System-Specific Physiology
System-Specific Assessments
System-Specific Labs and Diagnostic Procedures

A
Analysis of Concepts

F
First Do Priority Nursing Interventions
First Do Medications

E
Evaluation of Expected Outcomes

T
Trend for Potential Complications

Y
You Must Manage Care to Prevent "RISK" to the Client

Reference: National Council of State Boards of Nursing, Inc. (NCSBN) 2015

RISK

A structure for prioritizing Management and Safety NCLEX® Activities. Directions: *Please complete on your client assignment. Turn in to clinical instructor* _____.

R — Room Assignments, Recognize limitations of staff, Restraint safety, Risk for falls, Receive or give report

I — Identify trends, Infection control, Identification of client, Identify accuracy of orders, Informed consent, Interdisciplinary Team Collaboration

S — Skin breakdown, Safe equipment, Scope of Practice for delegation

K — Know Standards of Practice, Know how to document, Know how to prepare for transfer, discharge, Know how to teach and incorporate health-promotion standards

Reference: National Council of State Boards of Nursing, Inc. (NCSBN) 2015

AIDES

A structure for prioritizing Pharmacology NCLEX® Activities. Directions: *Please complete on ___ of your priority medications. Turn in to clinical instructor _____.*

NAME OF DRUG: BRAND _____ GENERIC _____

CLASSIFICATION: _____ REFERENCE USED _____

A Action of medication:

Administration of medication. Dosage ordered_____

How to administer:

Assessment:

Adverse Effects. List significant ones:

Accuracy/Appropriateness of order. Is it indicated based on client's condition, known allergies, drug-drug or drug-food interactions? If not, what action did you take?

I Interactions (Drug-Drug, Food-Drug):

Identify priority plan prior to giving drug (i.e., vital signs, labs, allergies, etc.):

Identify priority plan after giving drug:

D Desired outcomes of the drug:

Discharge teaching—Administration considerations for client and family:

Documentation:

E Evaluate client's response to medication:

S Safety (client identification, risk for falls, vital sign assessments):

Safe and controlled environment for handling and maintaining medicine:

Reference: National Council of State Boards of Nursing, Inc. (NCSBN) 2015

ENGAGING THE LEARNER ACTIVITIES

STUDENT-CENTERED LEARNING ACTIVITIES
LINKED TO PROFESSIONAL AND NCLEX® STANDARDS

Resources Needed for Activities	*Concepts Made Insanely Easy for Clinical Nursing* (Manning & Zager, 2014); *The Eight-Step Approach for Teaching Clinical Nursing* (Zager, Manning & Herman, 2017); *Medical Surgical Nursing Concepts Made Insanely Easy* (Manning & Zager, 2014)	*Concepts Made Insanely Easy for Clinical Nursing* (Manning & Zager, 2014); *The Eight-Step Approach for Student Clinical Success* (Zager, Manning & Herman, 2017); *Medical Surgical Nursing Concepts Made Insanely Easy* (Manning & Zager, 2014)
Standards	**Faculty Instructions**	**Student Instructions**

Management of Care
 	
Prioritize the delivery of client care.
	Trending for Potential Complications
	
	1. Ask students to identify potential complications with their assigned client.
	
	   a. What system-specific assessments would be a priority?
	
	   b. If they see a trend, what other assessments would provide additional information (i.e., VS, client behavior, labs, medication interactions, etc.).
	
	   c. What are the trends in the clinical findings (i.e., clinical results from the day before or during the clinical day)?
	
	   d. Compare and contrast the findings to the clinical norms or the client's normal.
	
	   e. What clinical findings would need to be reported to the assigned nurse and/or the healthcare provider?
		Trending for Potential Complications
		
		1. Based on your assigned client, what are the potential complications?
		
		   a. What system-specific assessments would be a priority?
		
		   b. If you see a trend, what other assessments would provide additional information?
		
		   c. What are the trends in the clinical findings?
		
		   d. Compare and contrast the findings to the clinical norms or the client's normal.
		
		   e. What clinical findings would need to be reported to the assigned nurse and/or the healthcare provider?

Safe and Effective Care Environment
 	
Apply principles of infection control (i.e., hand hygiene, room assignment, isolation, etc.).
	RISK to the Client—Infection Control
	(Refer to Chapter 23, *Medical Surgical Nursing Concepts Made Insanely Easy*)
	
	2. On index cards, provide client scenarios with different infections requiring specific care to pairs of students. Have the personal protective equipment (PPE) available to use.
	
	   a. Provide student pairs index cards of clients with different infections from different organisms that require care. They must choose the appropriate PPE for the care to be provided to the client (i.e., pertussis, HIV, pneumonia from MRSA, with rubella x 3 days, TB, etc.).
	
	   b. Provide student pairs 4 index cards and have them determine which two of 4 clients can share a room. Example of clients include post-op appendectomy with MRSA; hospital acquired C. diff; hepatitis, and MRSA from a traumatic injury to the right leg. The answer: the two MRSA clients.
		RISK to the Client—Infection Control
		(Refer to Chapter 23, *Medical Surgical Nursing Concepts Made Insanely Easy*)
		
		2. Based on the clients:
		
		   a. Choose the PPE needed for the care you will provide to your client indicated on the index card.
		
		   b. Which two of your 4 clients indicated on the index cards can share a room, a client post-op appendectomy with MRSA, a client with hospital acquired C. diff, a client admitted with hepatitis, or a client with MRSA from a traumatic injury to the right leg?

NOTES

References

Agency for Healthcare Research and Quality (AHRQ). Retrieved from http://www.ahrq.gov/, November 10, 2016.

Agency for Healthcare Research and Quality (2015). Medication errors. Retrieved from https://psnet.ahrq.gov/primers/primer/23/medication-errorsc.

Blum, C.A., Borglund, S., & Parcells, D. (2010). High-fidelity nursing simulation: Impact on student self-confidence and clinical competence. *International Journal of Nursing Education Scholarship, 7*(article 18), Retrieved from https://www.ncbi.nlm.nih.gov/pubmed/20597857.

Center for Disease Control (2015). Growth chart training. Retrieved from http://www.cdc.gov/nccdphp/dnpao/growthcharts/.

Dreifuerst, K.T. (2009). The essentials of debriefing in simulation learning: A concept analysis. Nursing Education Perspectives. 30(2), 109-114.

Dreifuerst, K.T. (2012). Using debriefing for meaning learning to foster development of clinical reasoning in simulation. Journal of Nursing Education. June 51(6), 326-333.

Hayden, J.K., Smiley, R.A., Alexander, M., Kardong-Edgren, S., & Jeffries, P.R. (2014). The NCSBN national simulation study: A longitudinal, randomized, controlled study replacing clinical hours with simulation in prelicensure nursing education. *Journal of Nursing Regulation. 5,* 1–66.

Herman, J., Manning, L., & Zager, L. (2011). The eight step approach to teaching clinical nursing. Duluth, GA: ICAN Publishing, Inc.

Herman, J. W. (2008). Creative teaching strategies for the nurse educator. Philadelphia, PA: F.A. Davis Company.

Hughes, R.G. (Ed) (2008). Patient Safety & Quality: An evidence-based handbook for nurses. (Prepared with support from the Robert Wood Johnson Foundation.) AHRQ Publication No. 08-0043. Rockville, MD: Agency for Healthcare Research and Quality; April 2008.

Institute for Safe Medication (ISMP). Retrieved from http://www.ismp.org/, November 16, 2016.

International Nursing Association for Clinical Simulation and Learning (INACSL). INACSL Standards of Best Practice: SimulationSM. Retrieved from http://www.inacsl.org/i4a/pages/index.cfm?pageid=3407, November 8, 2016.

Jefferies, P.R., & Clochesy, J.M. (2012). Clinical simulations: An experiential, student-centered pedagogical approach. In D. M. Billings and J.A. Halstead (Eds). Teaching in nursing: A guide for faculty (4th ed., pp 352-368). St. Louis, MO: Elsevier Health Sciences.

Jefferies, P.R., Dreifuerst, K.T., Kardon-Edgren, S., & Hayden, J. (2015). Faculty development when initialing simulation programs: Lessons learned from the National Simulation Study. Journal of Nursing Regulation, 5(4), 17-23.

Jefferies, P.R., & Rogers, K.J. (2102). Theoretical framework for simulation design. In P.R. Jeffries (Ed.), Simulation in nursing education: From conceptualization to evaluation (2nd ed., pp 25-41). New York, NY: National League for Nursing.

Kaufer, D. (2016). Neuroscience and how students learn. Graduate Student Instructor Teaching and Resource Center, How Students Learn Series, University of California Berkley. Retrieved from http://gsi.berkeley.edu/gsi-guide-contents/learning-theory-research/neuroscience .

Koharchik, L. (2014). Starting a job as adjunct clinical instructor. *American Journal of Nursing,* 114(8), p. 57-60.

Koharchnik, L, Caputi, L., Robb, M., & Culleiton, A. L. (2015). Fostering clinical reasoning in nursing students (2015). *American Journal of Nursing,* 115(1), 58-61.

Koharchnik, L, Weideman, Y. L., Walters, C. A., & Hardy, E. (2015). Evaluating nursing students' clinical performance. *American Journal of Nursing*, 115(10), 64-67.

Lioce L., Meakim, C.H., Fey, M.K., Chmil, J.V., Mariani, B., & Alinier, G. (2015). Standards of best practice: Simulation standard IX: Simulation design. *Clinical Simulation in Nursing*, 11(6), 309-315, Retrieved from http://dx.doi.org/10.1016/j.ecns.2015.03.005.

Manning, L. & Rayfield, S. (2016). Nursing made insanely easy, Duluth, GA: ICAN Publishing, Inc.

Manning, L. & Rayfield, S. (2017). Pharmacology made insanely easy. Duluth, GA: ICAN Publishing, Inc.

Manning, L. & Zager, L. (2014). Concepts made insanely easy for clinical nursing. Duluth, GA: ICAN Publishing, Inc.

Manning, L. & Zager, L. (2014). Medical surgical nursing concepts made insanely easy! A new approach to prioritization, Duluth, GA: ICAN Publishing, Inc.

Meakim, C., Boese, T., Decker, S., Franklin, A. E., Gloe, D., Lioce, L., Sando, C. R., & Borum, J. C. (2013). Standards of best practice: Simulation standard I: Terminology. *Clinical Simulation in Nursing*, 9(6S), S3-S11, Retrieved from http://dx.doi.org/10.1016/j.ecns.2013.04.001.

National Council of State Boards of Nursing. (NCSBN) 2014. RN Practice Analysis: Linking the NCLEX-RN® Examination to practice U.S. and Canada (Volume 62) January 2015.

National League for Nursing Simulation Innovation Resource Center (NLN-SIRC) (2013). SIRC glossary, Retrieved from http://sirc.nln.org/mod/glossary/view.php?id=183&mode=&hook=ALL&sortkey=&sortorder=&fullsearch=0&page=1.

National Patient Safety Goals (2017). 2017 Hospital national patient safety goals. Retrieved from https://www.jointcommission.org/assets/1/6/2017_NPSG_HAP_ER.pdf, January 12, 2017.

Nevid, J. (2011). Teaching the millennials. Retrieved from http://www.psychologicalscience.org/publications/observer/2011/may-june-11/teaching-the-millennials.html.

Penn, B.K. (Ed) (2008). Mastering the teaching role: A guide for nurse educators, Philadelphia, PA: F.A. Davis.

Pesut, D., & Herman, J.A., (1999). Clinical reasoning: The art and science of critical and creative thinking, Albany, NY: Delmar Publishing.

Quality and Safety Education for Nurses (QSEN). Retrieved from http://qsen.org/, November 22, 2016.

Reid, C. & Raleigh, R. (2013). Where to find simulations free. Retrieved from https://www.scribd.com/document/299632811/Where-to-Find-Simulation-Scenarios.

Simulation for Society in Healthcare 2016. Retrieved from http://www.ssih.org/About-Simulation, November 7, 2016.

Walls, C. (2006). The multitasking generation. Retrieved from http://www.time.com/time/archive/preview/0,10987,1174696,00.html.

Waxman, K. T. (2010). The development of evidence-based clinical simulation scenarios: Guidelines for nurse educators. *Journal of Nursing Education*, 49(1), 29-35.

Williams, A. (2015). Move over, millennials, here comes generation Z. Retrieved from http://www.nytimes.com/2015/09/20/fashion/move-over-millennials-here-comes-generation-z.html?_r=0.

World Health Organiztion (2010). National Center for Growth Statistics. Retrieved from https://cdc.gov/growthcharts/index.htm.

URLs for Simulation Scenarios, References and Scenario Design
http://www.sim-central.com/documents/scenarios.pdf
http://healthysimulation.com/5689/free-medical-simulation-scenarios/
http://healthysimulation.com/1947/more-free-nursing-simulation-scenarios/
http://sirc.nln.org/login/index.php
http://www.ksbn.org/education/Scenario/SimulationScenarioLibrary.htm
http://qsen.org/teaching-strategies/simulation/scenarios/
http://www.nursingsimulation.org/article/S1876-1399(15)00025-0/references

Index

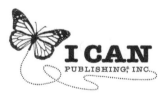
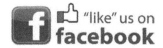